Improving Quality of Life for Individuals with Cerebral Palsy through Treatment of Gait Impairment

Clinics in Developmental Medicine

Improving Quality of Life for Individuals with Cerebral Palsy through Treatment of Gait Impairment: International Cerebral Palsy Function and Mobility Symposium

Edited by

Tom F Novacheck

Pediatric Orthopedic Surgeon; Associate Medical Director,
Gillette Children's Specialty Healthcare,
St. Paul, MN, USA.
Professor, Department of Orthopedics,
University of Minnesota

Michael H Schwartz

Clinical Scientist,
Gait and Motion Analysis Research,
Gillette Children's Specialty Healthcare,
St. Paul, MN, USA.
Professor, Department of Orthopedics,
University of Minnesota

2020
Mac Keith Press

© 2020 Mac Keith Press

Managing Director: Ann-Marie Halligan
Senior Publishing Manager: Sally Wilkinson
Publishing Co-ordinator: Lucy White

The views and opinions expressed herein are those of the authors and do not necessarily represent those of the publisher.

First published in this edition in 2020 by Mac Keith Press
2nd Floor, Rankin Building, 139–143 Bermondsey Street, London, SE1 3UW

British Library Cataloguing-in-Publication data
A catalogue record for this book is available from the British Library

Cover illustration modified from Bittmann MF, Lenhart RL, Schwartz MH, Novacheck TF, Hetzel S, Thelen DG (2018)
How does patellar tendon advancement alter the knee extensor mechanism in children treated for crouch gait? Gait Posture. 64 248–254, with permission from Elsevier.
Cover designer: Marten Sealby

ISBN: 978-1-911612-41-4

Typeset by Helena Loy

Contents

Author Appointments

Jon R Davids Assistant Chief of Orthopaedic Surgery; Medical Director Motion Analysis Laboratory, Shriners Hospitals for Children-NCA; Ben Ali Chair in Pediatric Orthopaedics, Department of Orthopaedic Surgery, University of California Davis, Sacramento, CA, USA.

Kaat Desloovere Doctor, Clinical Motion Analysis Laboratory, University Hospital Pellenberg, UZ Leuven; Professor, Department of Rehabilitation Sciences, Faculty of Kinesiology and Rehabilitation Sciences, KU Leuven, Pellenberg, Belgium.

Thomas Dreher Professor, Chief of Paediatric Orthopaedics, Balgrist University Hospital, Zurich, Switzerland.

Anahid Ebrahimi Research Associate, Department of Mechanical Engineering, University of Wisconsin-Madison, Madison, WI, USA.

Andrew G Georgiadis Pediatric Orthopaedic Surgeon; Director, James R. Gage Center for Gait and Motion Analysis, Gillette Children's Specialty Healthcare, St. Paul; Assistant Professor, Orthopaedic Surgery, University of Minnesota, Minneapolis, MN, USA.

H Kerr Graham Professor of Orthopaedic Surgery, University of Melbourne; Director, Hugh Williamson Gait Laboratory, Royal Children's Hospital, Melbourne, Australia.

Jason J Howard Pediatric Orthopedic Surgeon, Division of Cerebral Palsy, Department of Orthopedic Surgery, Nemours/Alfred I. duPont Hospital for Children, Wilmington, DE, USA.

Rick Lieber Chief Scientific Officer, Shirley Ryan AbilityLab; Professor of Physical Medicine and Rehabilitation, Feinberg School of Medicine, Northwesten University; Senior Research Career Scientist, Department of Veteran affairs, Rehabilitation Research & Developement, Chicago, IL, USA.

Warren A Marks Medical Director, Movement Disorders and Neurorehabilitation; Medical Director, Motion Analysis Laboratory, Cook Children's Medical Center, Fort Worth, Texas, USA.

Unni G Narayanan Professor, Departments of Surgery & Rehabilitation Sciences, Division of Orthopaedic Surgery, University of Toronto; Senior Associate Scientist, Child Health Evaluative Sciences Program, The Hospital for Sick Children, Toronto, Canada.

Tom F Novacheck Pediatric Orthopedic Surgeon; Associate Medical Director, Gillette Children's Specialty Healthcare, St. Paul, MN, USA. Professor, Department of Orthopedics, University of Minnesota.

Morgan Sangeux Research Fellow, The University of Melbourne, The Murdoch Children's Research Institute, Melbourne, Australia.

Michael H Schwartz Clinical Scientist, Gait and Motion Analysis Research, Gillette Children's Specialty Healthcare, St. Paul, MN, USA. Professor, Department of Orthopedics, University of Minnesota

Benjamin J Shore   Associate Professor in Orthopedic Surgery; Co-Director, Cerebral Palsy and Spasticity Center, Boston Childrens Hospital, Harvard Medical School, Boston, MA, USA.

Adam P Shortland   Consultant Clinical Scientist, Paediatric Neurosciences, Evelina Children's Hospital, Guy's & St Thomas' Foundation NHS Trust; Reader in Clinical Biomechanics, School of Biomedical Engineering and Imaging Sciences, King's College London, London, UK.

Katherine M Steele   Associate Professor, Mechanical Engineering, University of Washington, Seattle, USA.

Kristina Tedroff   Associate Professor, Neuropediatric Unit, Department of Women's and Children's Health, Karolinska Institutet; Consultant Pediatric Neurologist, Astrid Lindgren Children's Hospital, Karolinska University Hospital, Stockholm, Sweden.

Darryl G Thelen   John Bollinger Chair of Mechanical Engineering; Bernard A and Frances M Weideman Professor, University of Wisconsin, Madison, WI, USA.

Tim Theologis   Consultant Orthopaedic Surgeon, Oxford University Hospitals; Senior Clinical Lecturer, University of Oxford; Research Professor, Oxford Brooks University, Oxford, UK.

Marjolein van der Krogt   Amsterdam UMC, Vrije Universiteit Amsterdam, Department of Rehabilitation Medicine, Amsterdam Movement Sciences, Amsterdam, the Netherlands.

Preface

The genesis for this symposium was a Congenital Hemiplegia Think Tank organized by Dr Brian Neville in Cambridge England in the 1990's. Attending that meeting was a unique experience. Learning much from speakers with different focus, points of view, and ways of thinking, enlightened my naïve orthopedic point of view. I spoke about surgical treatment of gait problems. I was surprised that some attendees posed the question 'why should we do that?'. From their point of view, all individuals with hemiplegic CP ambulate in a very functional way even in the community with little to no assistance. At that time, it did not occur to me that these anatomical problems that affect the gait patterns for individuals with hemiplegic cerebral palsy (CP) might not warrant treatment. The publication from that symposium was also published by Mac Keith Press in 2000.

The uniqueness of that experience and the impact that it had on me led to discussions with Mike Schwartz two years ago about organizing a similarly designed conference. Mike and I have functioned in a dyadic model (clinician & scientist) over the past 23 years in the Center for Gait and Motion Analysis at Gillette Children's Specialty Healthcare. This experience led us to design a similar symposium but in this case pairing clinicians and scientists to discuss the current state of knowledge working at the border of what we know and what we don't. We undertook a fundraising effort with the Gillette Children's Specialty Healthcare Foundation supported by a steering committee made up of an engaged group of parents of adolescents and young adults with CP.

Invitees were recognized experts in CP with whom we had some prior relationship. Presentations were purposefully short to allow abundant time for debate and discussion. The symposium 'International Cerebral Palsy Function & Mobility Symposium: Improving Quality of Life for Individuals with Cerebral Palsy through Treatment of Gait Impairment' was held 11th to 13th December 2019 in Banff, Canada. We worked in the mornings and played in the afternoons! Because the ultimate goal of this symposium (and the chapters herein) was to help establish a framework to guide research efforts for the next years, it was our intention to publish this as quickly as possible.

We recognize that this is far from a comprehensive representation of all topics by all experts. First of all, this book focuses on gait and mobility which is but one aspect of wellbeing of an individual with CP in adulthood. Cognitive factors and upper extremity function are better predictors of success in psychosocial wellbeing, relationships, employment, and financial stability.

This work is meant to challenge long-held assumptions. It is meant to explore the current state of research, testing, and treatment. We asked the participants to not only be objective, but also to provide expert opinion. As such, you will notice that the authors present different views. The debates at the symposium were vigorous. Disagreements, different points of view, and lack of clarity were purposefully not edited out of the chapters. We did not strive to create consensus amongst the authors in this publication. It is our goal to allow you to engage in this richness at the intersection of expert opinion and science. By doing so, we hope that it stimulates your own scientific exploration. We unified the disparate topics using the common format of bulleted key points and objectives at the beginning of each chapter. If you find yourself wondering what happened during the debates, you will find your answers in the two bulleted lists at the end of each chapter.

We are very grateful to Rachel Wobschall of the Gillette Children's Foundation for all the work that she did to develop the energy and financial support for this meeting. We thank Amy Schall for her apt organizational skills as we planned for and executed this meeting. We recognize and acknowledge that if it weren't for Gillette Children's, Dr James R Gage, and the staff of the Center for Gait and Motion Analysis at Gillette, we could not have done this. We thank our generous donors without whom this symposium would not have happened:

- Anonymous
- Jim and Mary Gage
- Linda Hallman, DDS, PhD and Mike Freeman
- Perry and Sandra MacDonald
- Mac Keith Press
- McGough Construction
- Advanced Mechanical Technology Inc (AMTI).

And, we thank you for your interest in this work and your efforts to understand the lives and challenges of individuals with CP.

Tom F Novacheck, MD
March 2020

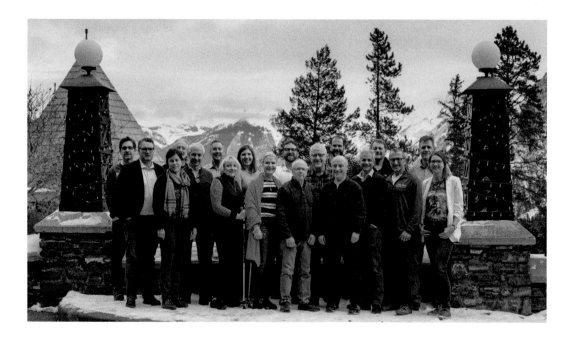

Acknowledgements

Jason J Howard, H Kerr Graham, and Adam P Shortland acknowledge Dr Robert Akins, Alfred I. duPont Hospital for Children (Wilmington, DE, USA), for reviewing the manuscript and providing feedback.

H Kerr Graham acknowledges support from NHMRC CP-Achieve Grant.

Lever Arm Dysfunction
Improving Care Requires Greater Knowledge of Early Development and Long-Term Consequences

Katherine M Steele and Andrew G Georgiadis

KEY POINTS

- Altered bone morphology is common in cerebral palsy (CP), affecting individuals' abilities to effectively transfer forces and move in the world.
- Bone morphology provides a window into the history of an individual's growth, development, and activity.
- Orthopaedic surgery alters alignment and current standards seek to restore alignment within normative ranges.

OPPORTUNITIES

- Advancements in imaging provide greater precision for safely quantifying and monitoring morphology.
- Early detection and monitoring can enhance our knowledge of how altered bone morphology develops and improve our ability to prevent impairments that impact function.
- Long-term follow-up is necessary to understand the impacts of altered morphology and current interventions on mobility, participation, and quality of life for adults with CP.

A lever arm is defined as the perpendicular distance between an axis and a force's line of action (Fig. 1.1). Within the musculoskeletal system, a muscle produces force, and the resulting joint moments and movement are dependent upon its lever arm (Bowen 1912; Fenn 1938; Elftman 1939). For children with cerebral palsy (CP), altered skeletal anatomy often reduces the length of important lever arms in the lower extremity, contributing to gait impairments by diminishing a muscle's moment-generating capacity. This has been termed lever arm dysfunction (LAD). LAD provides a useful framework for understanding how altered alignment of the lower-extremities can influence movement and function.

For over two decades, consideration of LAD has been important in the evaluation and treatment of CP (Gage 1991; Gage and Schwartz 2001; Gage and Schwartz 2004). The most common sources of

LAD among people with CP are due to femoral anteversion, tibial torsion, and foot deformity (Wren et al. 2005). Bone deformities can contribute to LAD at multiple levels (Fig. 1.1). For example, femoral anteversion can affect hip movement by reducing the lever arm of the gluteus medius muscle, requiring greater muscle force to achieve the required hip abduction moment and further increasing internal rotation (Arnold et al. 1997; Delp et al. 1999; Gage and Novacheck 2001). Femoral anteversion also alters the orientation of the leg, which can induce LAD at other levels. Internal rotation of the foot, caused by femoral anteversion or other malalignments, affects the lever arm of the ground reaction force relative to both the knee and ankle. This altered alignment increases the demand on the ankle plantar flexors to extend the ankle, while also reducing the extension moment at the knee – commonly referred to as the plantar flexion-knee extension couple (Gage et al. 1987; DeLuca, 1991; Schwartz and Lakin 2003). This example illustrates how altered alignment of one segment can lead to LAD across all lower extremity joints and the complex interactions that we must consider to evaluate walking dynamics among people with CP.

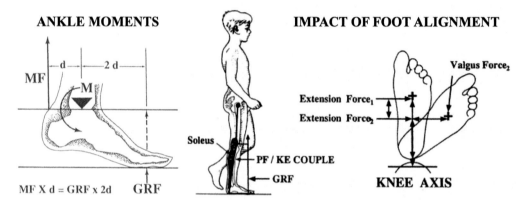

Figure 1.1 Lever arm dysfunction (LAD) can arise from skeletal alignment, posture (e.g. crouch gait), or altered joint function (e.g. hip subluxation or pes valgus). A lever arm is defined as the perpendicular distance between a point and a force's line of action. In the musculoskeletal system, lever arms can be used to evaluate the moment-generating capacity of muscles, as well as the impact of the ground reaction force (GRF) or other external forces (e.g. orthoses) on joint moments. For example, the lever arm (d) of the plantar flexors (MF) about the ankle might be half that of the lever arm (2d) of the GRF. Rotation of the leg, caused by femoral anteversion, tibial torsion, or posture is one common cause of LAD in CP. Rotation of the foot can reduce the knee extension moment of the GRF, reducing the magnitude of the plantar flexion-knee extension couple (PF/KE Couple) in stance. Reprinted from Novacheck and Gage 2007 with permission from Springer Nature.

Understanding altered bony alignment and LAD is critical to improving care and function of people with CP. Bone morphology can provide clinicians with a snapshot of the cumulative effects of the complex neuromuscular and musculoskeletal changes after neurological injury early in development (Carter et al. 1996). While CP is caused by an injury to the brain near the time of birth, the secondary effects on musculoskeletal development are important to understand and improve movement (Graham and Selber 2003). Bones generally grow and remodel in response to the forces and demands experienced in daily life, a principle known as Wolff's Law (Frost 1994). Thus, a child's bone morphology reflects their activity, movement patterns, and muscle activity over their lifetime. Bones give a summative snapshot of their movement and function. This is especially relevant in early development as, according to the Heuter-Volkmann principle, the distractive or compressive loads on the growth plate dictate longitudinal growth (Arkin and Katz 1956; Swanson et al. 1963; Leveau and Bernhardt 1984). Using the example of femoral alignment, typically developing children have roughly 40° of anteversion at birth due to positioning in the womb (Felts 1954; Somerville 1957).

During development, the femur remodels and femoral anteversion decreases to 10° to 15° by adolescence, with the greatest remodeling occurring in the first four years of life (Shands Jr and Steele 1958; Crane 1959; Fabry et al. 1973). Delayed mobility and altered movement patterns in CP are thought to impact this remodeling and contribute to excessive femoral anteversion (Robin et al. 2008). Similar effects on the growth and development of the tibia and foot are thought to contribute to excessive tibial torsion and foot deformities commonly observed in CP (O'Connell et al. 1998; Rethlefsen et al. 2006).

Our understanding of LAD has had a strong influence on the design of current interventions used to improve gait for children with CP, especially in orthopaedic surgery and orthotic design (Vankoski et al. 2000; Novacheck and Gage 2007). A core tenet of multilevel surgery (MLS) is to correct alignment, reducing the impacts of LAD and improving walking function. Derotational osteotomies, guided growth, foot procedures, and other surgeries seek to align the leg within normative ranges (Hoffer et al. 1985). These surgeries are effective at correcting alignment, but the impact on walking function is highly variable. As an example, historically about 40% of children with bilateral CP at one institution who received gait analysis for surgical consideration underwent a femoral derotation osteotomy (FDO) (Fig. 1.2.) The osteotomy significantly reduced anteversion at their post-operative gait analysis (*–31.4°, n=137*) compared to peers with bilateral CP who did not undergo the procedure (*–2.4°, n=207*). However, changes in walking function were highly variable. About half of the children who received an FDO had clinically significant improvements in kinematics (change in Gait Deviation Index >5).

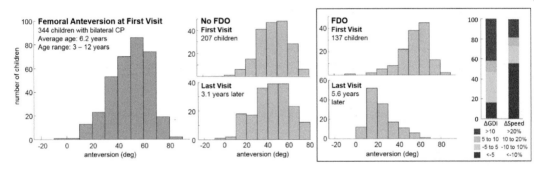

Figure 1.2 Increased femoral anteversion is common among children with cerebral palsy (CP) referred for gait analysis. Historically, the femoral anteversion at the first visit was 47° for children with bilateral CP at their first gait analysis. Femoral derotation osteotomy (FDO) is used to align the femur and correct internal rotation during gait. Among children with bilateral CP who had multiple gait analyses, 40% underwent an FDO and had a significant reduction in femoral anteversion at their follow-up gait analysis (31.4° reduction in anteversion). In comparison, children with bilateral CP who did not receive an FDO – because the procedure was not recommended or other procedures were selected – experienced minimal changes in anteversion between gait analyses (2.4° reduction in anteversion), suggesting that femoral anteversion was relatively stable with age for this group. Most children who received an FDO received other procedures as part of a multilevel surgery, which makes determining the direct impacts of FDO on gait challenging. There was large variability in changes in gait kinematics (e.g. Gait Deviation Index) and walking speed (e.g. dimensionless speed to account for growth) between individuals who received an FDO. Images courtesy of James R. Gage Center for Gait and Motion Analysis at Gillette Children's Specialty Healthcare.

While LAD has provided a framework to evaluate the biomechanics of altered gait and inspired new interventions, numerous gaps limit our understanding and treatment of gait for children with CP. The following sections outline three such gaps that we view as critical for improving function: (1) tracking early development, (2) understanding foot morphology, and (3) examining the long-term consequences of LAD. For each, we discuss the current state of knowledge and needs for future research. We also highlight a few opportunities that we believe can amplify these efforts and further advance care for children with CP.

Critical Gaps

EARLY DEVELOPMENT

While bone growth and development have been well-characterized for typically developing children, early bone growth among children with CP is not documented. Accurate measurements of bone morphology are typically not taken for children with CP until they are referred for gait analysis or orthopaedic surgery at 5 or more years of age. A subset of children with CP undergo radiographic hip surveillance starting at 2 or 3 years of age, but even these evaluations focus on the hip and pelvis with limited information about the alignment and growth of the leg (Dobson et al. 2002). As a result, we know that excessive femoral anteversion, tibial torsion, and foot deformity are common in children with CP, but when or how these deformities develop and whether they could be prevented is unknown.

The basic science underlying our understanding of bone growth is also unknown for CP. While Wolff's Law and the Heuter-Volkmann principle provide a framework to describe bone growth and remodeling during typical development, to what extent these principles extend to children with CP remains unknown (Bertram and Swartz 1991; Yaşar et al. 2018). Extensive prior research has demonstrated that the basic metabolic, mechanosensory, and material properties of bone and muscle are altered in CP (Henderson et al. 2002; Wingert et al. 2009; Peterson et al. 2012). We know that CP muscle does not grow or respond to mechanical cues like typically developing muscle, resulting in long sarcomeres and other structural differences that impact muscle force and function (see Chapter 7 [Mathewson and Lieber 2015]). Assuming that CP bone grows and responds to daily demands like typically developing bone could be a flawed or incomplete theory. A few studies have shown that computational models (e.g. finite element models) that follow Wolff's Law predict bone deformities like femoral anteversion observed in CP when the altered loading of CP gait are applied (Shefelbine and Carter 2004, Carriero et al. 2011), but assumptions of bone growth and development need to be carefully examined for children with CP.

The Foot

The foot acts as our ultimate lever, transferring the forces we produce to the ground so we can move and explore our world. Unfortunately, the foot is also very complex – with 26 bones, 20 internal muscles, numerous polyarticular tendons, and complex passive structures – even understanding the form and function of a typically developing foot remains challenging. Describing the foot as a lever is itself an approximation, where the net effect of this complex structure across multiple joints is combined to evaluate walking dynamics.

Children with CP present with a wide array of foot deformities (Baker and Hill 1964; Bennet et al. 1982; O'Connell et al. 1998). Equinoplanovalgus, equinovarus, and equinocavovarus are among the most common. Each of these deformities has a different effect on the alignment of the foot, the transfer of forces, and the subsequent impact on walking dynamics. Further, the developmental trajectory and long-term prognosis of each deformity is thought to be unique. Typically developing children have a flat foot as toddlers, which develops into an arch by 4 years of age (Gould et al. 1989). Clinicians often assume similar developmental trajectories for young children with CP, but with the expectation that the observed deformities in some children will not correct with development and require intervention (Wenger et al. 1989). Shoes and orthoses add an extra layer of complexity, whereby the immediate and long-term effects on walking function and foot shape are poorly understood (Rao and Joseph 1992). Detailing the structure, development, and dynamics of the foot among children with CP is critical to provide a solid foundation for walking function.

Extensive research has attempted to elucidate foot dynamics during gait for children with CP. The most common method has been developing multi-segment foot models for clinical gait analysis (Carson et al.

2001; Stebbins et al. 2006; Deschamps et al. 2012; Leardini et al. 2019). Early gait analyses often relied on simple marker sets (e.g. single markers on the toe, heel, and malleoli) that largely captured 'ankle' motion but were prone to errors by ignoring motion within the foot. For example, ignoring motion about the metatarsophalangeal joint or mid-foot collapse would lead to incorrect estimates of ankle angle during stance (Kim and Kipp 2019). Multi-segment foot models overcome some of these challenges, but properly placing these markers with respect to bony landmarks and skin movement during walking make their accuracy and interpretation challenging (Shultz et al. 2011). Even when radiographs are used to determine the placement of markers with respect to underlying bones (Saraswat et al. 2012), understanding the movement of these markers during gait and the appropriate coordinate systems to describe foot motion is difficult. Beyond bony alignment, very little is known about the passive structures of the foot and how they might be altered in CP. Because of these challenges, many of our biomechanical models and analyses are based upon highly-simplified models that assume a rigid foot, or a few simplified segments. Multiple groups are working to develop improved foot and contact models (DeMers et al. 2017; Malaquias et al. 2017; Akrami et al. 2018), but often the appropriate morphology and mechanical properties to inform these models remain unknown. New methods and theory are critically needed to improve our understanding of the foot, the effect of foot deformities on gait, and the impact of shoes, orthoses, and other interventions.

Long-Term Consequences

The long-term consequences of LAD left untreated or with surgical correction, on function and quality of life remain unknown. Understanding the long-term effects of altered gait biomechanics on pain, joint degeneration, mobility, and participation are important to inform care and treatment planning (Opheim et al. 2013; Morgan and McGinley 2014). Over 60% of adults with CP experience a deterioration in walking function by 40 years of age (Opheim et al. 2009). Over 40% of adults with CP experience knee pain that impacts function in daily life (Jahnsen et al. 2004). We need to understand whether pain and function in adulthood are related to altered bone morphology or gait pattern, and if current treatments prevent or accelerate declines in mobility during adulthood.

Research in adults with CP to better understand these effects represents a critical unmet need. While children with CP have an integrated care team and receive regular therapy, there are fewer resources or trained clinicians for adults with CP (Binks et al. 2007). Only recently has the infrastructure been available to support long-term follow-up studies that evaluate walking function 10 years or more after childhood interventions. Returning to the example of femoral anteversion, recent work by Boyer and colleagues (Boyer et al. 2020) compared long-term outcomes among patients with CP who underwent proximal FDO and matched peers with CP who did not undergo this procedure. All participants were now over 25 years of age with a follow-up time of more than 13 years after their initial evaluation. As expected, femoral anteversion was significantly reduced after FDO and maintained at long-term follow-up. The group who did not undergo an FDO still had excessive femoral anteversion, suggesting natural development did not correct the excessive anteversion. Functionally, there were no differences between groups in hip rotation during stance or measures of pain or osteoarthritis. However, similar to prior studies of long-term outcomes (Brunner and Baumann 1997; Õunpuu et al. 2002; Dreher et al. 2012), these are still young adults, whom we hope are not faced with early joint pain or osteoarthritis. Whether procedures like FDO reduce contact forces (Passmore et al. 2018), prevent pain or osteoarthritis, and support lifetime mobility remain unknown. New techniques are needed to understand the long-term effects of LAD, as well as to provide options and guidance for adults with CP.

OPPORTUNITIES

While these gaps represent significant challenges, there are numerous advancements that we are confident will help bridge these gaps, support research, and accelerate clinical translation. Innovations in imaging provide unprecedented precision and access to techniques that will let us monitor bone morphology and foot function throughout the lifespan (Fig. 1.3). X-ray images and computed tomography (CT) scans have long been the standard to evaluate bone morphology, but both require significant radiation doses and can typically only be done under static conditions. Improvements in X-ray techniques, such as systems that integrate 2D X-ray scans with 3D-skeletal models from multiple angles (e.g. EOS Imaging System) can provide much more detailed and accurate measurements of bone alignment while standing or in other postures with significant reductions in radiation (Folinais et al. 2013; Sung et al. 2019). Similarly, biplane fluoroscopy uses two intersecting fluoroscopic video X-rays to capture synchronized stereo images with high temporal and spatial resolution. Combining these images with an individual's unique bone geometry from a CT scan can allow researchers to accurately track bone movement, including the bones of the feet, during walking or other movement (Iaquinto et al. 2014; Ito et al. 2017; Iaquinto et al. 2018). These imaging advancements will open new doors to improve our understanding of early bone growth, monitor long-term changes, and examine complexities of foot motion during dynamic activities. New techniques will still be required to use these techniques for research and clinical evaluations and connect bone morphology to neuromuscular function, but provide exciting opportunities to advance our field.

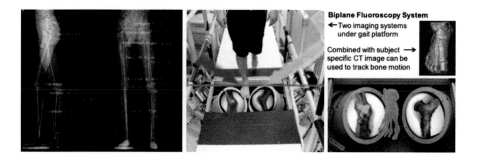

Figure 1.3 Advances in imaging can improve our ability to accurately measure and monitor bone growth and function in CP. (Left) Low-dose, multi-planar radiographic system, like the EOS system, lets clinicians measure and monitor the longitudinal and torsional alignment of the femur and tibia to inform treatment planning. The multi-planar measurements of bony anatomy are provided in separate reports, not pictured. (Right) Biplane fluoroscopy systems can image a part of the body, such as the foot, during walking to evaluate the alignment of bones, investigate how alignment impacts function, and evaluate the impact of orthoses or other assistive devices. Images courtesy of William Ledoux, Joseph Iaquinto, Eric Thorhauer, VA Puget Sound Center for Limb Loss & Mobility.

Over the past three decades, there has been an increase in the availability and use of registries and other clinical databases for people with CP (Cans et al. 2004). These registries have been critical for understanding long-term function and identifying gaps in current care pathways. However, these registries are still only available in a few locations and are largely limited to traditional clinical exams and surveys. These databases have not been connected to gait analyses or other quantitative measures of movement. We need to be able to expand current databases, easily connect and compare across sites, and triangulate with other data (e.g. surgical history, gait analysis, or activity levels from wearable sensors) to understand the impact of current interventions and support individuals with CP across their lifespan. Such databases could be used to address many of the gaps we identified for understanding bone alignment and LAD. For example, differences in surgical standards between locations can be used to evaluate matched groups who did or did not undergo a specific surgical procedure. Pooling data across clinical centers or countries also lets us examine and model growth trajectories (e.g. femoral anteversion) during childhood and adulthood, with or without treatment. Continuing to expand the breadth and access to these databases will provide powerful tools to support future care and quality of life of people with CP.

CONCLUSION

Evaluations of bone alignment and LAD have been cornerstones of our biomechanical and orthopaedic theory used to evaluate and improve gait for people with CP. New tools and techniques will help us better understand the development of these impairments, their impact on dynamic activities, and their long-term consequences. Several critical assumptions about bone growth and foot function need to be evaluated to determine whether they extend to people with CP. The next decades will hopefully bring new research and clinical practices that will enable clinicians to accurately predict and track musculoskeletal development, prevent the need for invasive procedures to correct altered morphology, and support mobility and participation throughout life for people with CP.

5-YEAR PRIORITIES

- **Track development:** Monitor morphology from early childhood to understand growth trajectories and examine factors (e.g. age of first steps) that influence early development.
- **Evaluate early interventions:** Evaluate the impact of early interventions (e.g. early prescription of orthoses or walkers) on bone alignment.
- **Delay intervention:** Delay orthopaedic procedures for ≥1 years to monitor changes in gait and bone morphology with natural growth.
- **Examine foot dynamics:** Use biplane fluoroscopy to evaluate foot dynamics for common CP foot deformities, including the impact of shoes, orthoses, and current surgical interventions.
- **Monitor mobility:** Use gait analysis, imaging, and wearable sensing to evaluate the effects of bone deformities and other impairments on mobility and participation for adults with CP.

FUTURE NEEDS

- **Foot theory:** Foundational knowledge for quantifying and evaluating dynamics of the foot for people with CP, including the interplay between altered bone morphology, muscle properties, passive tissues, and motor control.
- **Prevention:** Novel methods that can prevent bone deformities and LAD to avoid the need for orthopaedic surgery or other invasive procedures.
- **Prediction:** Models that can predict an individual's future growth and development given their unique morphology, motor control, and daily activity.

REFERENCES

Akrami M, Qian Z, Zou Z, Howard D, Nester CJ, Ren L (2018) Subject-specific finite element modelling of the human foot complex during walking: sensitivity analysis of material properties, boundary and loading conditions. *Biomech Model Mechanobiol* **17**: 559–576.

Arkin AM, Katz JF (1956) The effects of pressure on epiphyseal growth: the mechanism of plasticity of growing bone. *JBJS* **38**: 1056–1076.

Arnold AS, Komallu AV, Delp SL (1997) Internal rotation gait: a compensatory mechanism to restore abduction capacity decreased by bone deformity? *Developmental Medicine & Child Neurology* **39**: 40–44.

Baker LD, Hill LM (1964) Foot alignment in the cerebral palsy patient. *JBJS* **46**: 1–15.

Bennet GC, Rang M, Jones D (1982) Varus and valgus deformities of the foot in cerebral palsy. *Developmental Medicine & Child Neurology* **24**: 499–503.

Bertram JE, Swartz SM (1991) The 'law of bone transformation': a case of crying Wolff? *Biological Reviews* **66**: 245–273.

Binks JA, Barden WS, Burke TA, Young NL (2007) What do we really know about the transition to adult-centered health care? A focus on cerebral palsy and spina bifida. *Archives of physical medicine and rehabilitation* **88**: 1064–1073.

Bowen WP (1912) *Action of Muscles in Bodily Movement & Posture*. Michigan State Normal College: Nabu Press.

Boyer ER, Walt K, Munoz A, Healy M, Schwartz MH, Novacheck TF (2020) *Long-term outcomes of femoral derotation osteotomy in ambulatory individuals with cerebral palsy*. Virtual Conference 23–26 September 2020. Unpublished.

Brunner R, Baumann J (1997) Long-term effects of intertrochanteric varus-derotation osteotomy on femur and acetabulum in spastic cerebral palsy: an 11-to 18-year follow-up study. *Journal of Pediatric Orthopaedics* **17**: 585–591.

Cans C, Surman G, Mcmanus V, Coghlan D, Hensey O, Johnson A (2004) Cerebral palsy registries. *Seminars in pediatric neurology* **11**: 18–23.

Carriero A, Jonkers I, Shefelbine SJ (2011) Mechanobiological prediction of proximal femoral deformities in children with cerebral palsy. *Computer methods in biomechanics and biomedical engineering* **14**: 253–262.

Carson MC, Harrington ME, Thompson N, O'Connor JJ, Theologis TN (2001) Kinematic analysis of a multi-segment foot model for research and clinical applications: a repeatability analysis. *J Biomech* **34**: 1299–1307.

Carter D, Van der Meulen M, Beaupre G (1996) Mechanical factors in bone growth and development. *Bone* **18**: S5–S10.

Crane L (1959) Femoral torsion and its relation to toeing-in and toeing-out. *JBJS* **41**: 421–428.

Delp SL, Hess WE, Hungerford DS, Jones LC (1999) Variation of rotation moment arms with hip flexion. *Journal of biomechanics* **32**: 493–501.

Deluca PA (1991) The use of gait analysis and dynamic EMG in the assessment of the child with cerebral palsy. *Human Movement Science* **10**: 543–554.

Demers MS, Hicks JL, Delp SL (2017) Preparatory co-activation of the ankle muscles may prevent ankle inversion injuries. *J Biomech* **52**: 17–23.

Deschamps K, Staes F, Bruyninckx H et al. (2012) Repeatability in the assessment of multi-segment foot kinematics. *Gait Posture* **35**: 255–260.

Dobson F, Boyd R, Parrott J, Nattrass G, Graham H (2002) Hip surveillance in children with cerebral palsy: impact on the surgical management of spastic hip disease. *The Journal of bone and joint surgery. British volume* **84**: 720–726.

Dreher T, Wolf SI, Heitzmann D et al. (2012) Long-term outcome of femoral derotation osteotomy in children with spastic diplegia. *Gait Posture* **36**: 467–470.

Elftman H (1939) The function of muscles in locomotion. *American Journal of Physiology-Legacy Content* **125**: 357–366.

Fabry G, Macewen GD, Shands Jr A (1973) Torsion of the Femur: A follow-up study in normal and abnormal conditions. *JBJS* **55**: 1726–1738.

Felts WJ (1954) The prenatal development of the human femur. *American Journal of anatomy* **94**: 1–44.

Fenn W (1938) The mechanics of muscular contraction in man. *Journal of Applied Physics* **9**: 165–177.

Folinais D, Thelen P, Delin C, Radier C, Catonne Y, Lazennec J (2013) Measuring femoral and rotational alignment: EOS system versus computed tomography. *Orthopaedics & Traumatology: Surgery & Research* **99**: 509–516.

Frost HM (1994) Wolff's Law and bone's structural adaptations to mechanical usage: an overview for clinicians. *The Angle Orthodontist* **64**: 175–188.

Gage JR (1991) *Gait Analysis in Cerebral Palsy*. London: Mac Keith Press.

Gage JR, Novacheck TF (2001) An update on the treatment of gait problems in cerebral palsy. *Journal of Pediatric Orthopaedics Part B* **10**: 265–274.

Gage JR, Perry J, Hicks RR, Koop S, Werntz JR (1987) Rectus femoris transfer to improve knee function of children with cerebral palsy. *Developmental Medicine & Child Neurology* **29**: 159–166.

Gage JR, Schwartz MH (2001) Dynamic deformities and lever arm considerations. In: Paley D, editor, *Principles of Deformity*. Berlin: Springer.

Gage JR, Schwartz MH (2004) Pathological gait and lever-arm dysfunction. In: Gage JR, editor, *The Treatment of Gait Problems in Cerebral Palsy*. London: Mac Keith Press.

Gould N, Moreland M, Alvarez R, Trevino S, Fenwick J (1989) Development of the child's arch. *Foot & Ankle* **9**: 241–245.

Graham H, Selber P (2003) Musculoskeletal aspects of cerebral palsy. *Journal of Bone & Joint Surgery, British Volume* **85**: 157–166.

Henderson RC, Lark RK, Gurka MJ et al. (2002) Bone density and metabolism in children and adolescents with moderate to severe cerebral palsy. *Pediatrics* **110**: e5–e5.

Hoffer MM, Stein G, Koffman M, Prietto M (1985) Femoral varus-derotation osteotomy in spastic cerebral palsy. *The Journal of bone and joint surgery. American volume* **67**: 1229–1235.

Iaquinto JM, Kindig MW, Haynor DR et al. (2018) Model-based tracking of the bones of the foot: A biplane fluoroscopy validation study. *Comput Biol Med* **92**: 118–127.

Iaquinto JM, Tsai R, Haynor DR, Fassbind MJ, Sangeorzan BJ, Ledoux WR (2014) Marker-based validation of a biplane fluoroscopy system for quantifying foot kinematics. *Med Eng Phys* **36**: 391–396.

Ito K, Hosoda K, Shimizu M et al. (2017) Three-Dimensional Innate Mobility Of The Human Foot Bones Under Axial Loading Using Biplane X-Ray Fluoroscopy. *R Soc Open Sci* **4**: 171086.

Jahnsen R, Villien L, Aamodt G, Stanghelle JK, Holm I (2004) Musculoskeletal pain in adults with cerebral palsy compared with the general population. *J Rehabil Med,* **36**: 78–84.

Kim H, Kipp K (2019) Number of Segments Within Musculoskeletal Foot Models Influences Ankle Kinematics and Strains of Ligaments and Muscles. *J Orthop Res* **37**: 2231–2240.

Leardini A, Caravaggi P, Theologis T, Stebbins J (2019) Multi-segment foot models and their use in clinical populations. *Gait Posture* **69**: 50–59.

Leveau BF, Bernhardt DB (1984) Developmental biomechanics: effect of forces on the growth, development, and maintenance of the human body. *Physical Therapy* **64**: 1874–1882.

Malaquias TM, Silveira C, Aerts W et al. (2017) Extended foot-ankle musculoskeletal models for application in movement analysis. *Comput Methods Biomech Biomed Engin* **20**: 153–159.

Mathewson MA, Lieber RL (2015) Pathophysiology of muscle contractures in cerebral palsy. *Physical Medicine and Rehabilitation Clinics* **26**: 57–67.

Morgan P, Mcginley J (2014) Gait function and decline in adults with cerebral palsy: a systematic review. *Disability and rehabilitation* **36**: 1–9.

Novacheck TF, Gage JR (2007) Orthopedic management of spasticity in cerebral palsy. *Child's Nervous System* **23**: 1015–1031.

O'connell PA, D'souza L, Dudeney S, Stephens M (1998) Foot deformities in children with cerebral palsy. *Journal of Pediatric Orthopaedics* **18**: 743–747.

Opheim A, Jahnsen R, Olsson E, Stanghelle JK (2009) Walking function, pain, and fatigue in adults with cerebral palsy: a 7-year follow-up study. *Dev Med Child Neurol* **51**: 381–388.

Opheim A, Mcginley J, Olsson E, Stanghelle J, Jahnsen R (2013) Walking deterioration and gait analysis in adults with spastic bilateral cerebral palsy. *Gait Posture* **37**: 165–171.

Passmore E, Graham HK, Pandy MG, Sangeux M (2018) Hip-and patellofemoral-joint loading during gait are increased in children with idiopathic torsional deformities. *Gait Posture* **63**: 228–235.

Peterson MD, Gordon PM, Hurvitz EA, Burant CF (2012) Secondary muscle pathology and metabolic dysregulation in adults with cerebral palsy. *American Journal of Physiology-Endocrinology and Metabolism* **303**: E1085–E1093.

Rao UB, Joseph B (1992) The influence of footwear on the prevalence of flat foot. A survey of 2300 children. *The Journal of bone and joint surgery. British volume* **74**: 525–527.

Rethlefsen SA, Healy BS, Wren TA, Skaggs DL, Kay RM (2006) Causes of intoeing gait in children with cerebral palsy. *JBJS* **88**: 2175–2180.

Robin J, Graham HK, Selber P, Dobson F, Smith K, Baker R (2008) Proximal femoral geometry in cerebral palsy: a population-based cross-sectional study. *The Journal of bone and joint surgery. British volume* **90**: 1372–1379.

Saraswat P, Macwilliams BA, Davis RB (2012) A multi-segment foot model based on anatomically registered technical coordinate systems: method repeatability in pediatric feet. *Gait Posture* **35**: 547–555.

Schwartz M, Lakin G (2003) The effect of tibial torsion on the dynamic function of the soleus during gait. *Gait Posture* **17**: 113–118.

Shands Jr A, Steele MK (1958) Torsion of the femur: a follow-up report on the use of the Dunlap method for its determination. *JBJS* **40**: 803–816.

Shefelbine SJ, Carter DR (2004) Mechanobiological predictions of femoral anteversion in cerebral palsy. *Ann Biomed Eng* **32**: 297–305.

Shultz R, Kedgley AE, Jenkyn TR (2011) Quantifying skin motion artifact error of the hindfoot and forefoot marker clusters with the optical tracking of a multi-segment foot model using single-plane fluoroscopy. *Gait Posture* **34**: 44–48.

Somerville E (1957) Persistent foetal alignment of the hip. *The Journal of bone and joint surgery. British volume* **39**: 106–113.

Stebbins J, Harrington M, Thompson N, Zavatsky A, Theologis T (2006) Repeatability of a model for measuring multi-segment foot kinematics in children. *Gait Posture* **23**: 401–410.

Sung KH, Youn K, Chung CY et al. (2020) Development and Validation of a Mobile Application for Measuring Femoral Anteversion in Patients With Cerebral Palsy. *J Pediatr Orthop* **40**: e516–e521

Swanson AB, Greene Jr PW, Allis HD (1963) 13 Rotational Deformities of the Lower Extremity in Children and Their Clinical Significance. *Clinical Orthopaedics and Related Research* **27**: 157–175.

Vankoski SJ, Michaud S, Dias L (2000) External Tibial Torsion and the Effectiveness of the Solid Ankle–Foot Orthoses. *Journal of Pediatric Orthopaedics* **20**: 349–355.

Wenger DR, Mauldin D, Speck G, Morgan D, Lieber RL (1989) Corrective shoes and inserts as treatment for flexible flatfoot in infants and children. *JBJS* **71**: 800–810.

Wingert JR, Burton H, Sinclair RJ, Brunstrom JE, Damiano DL (2009) Joint-position sense and kinesthesia in cerebral palsy. *Archives of physical medicine and rehabilitation* **90**: 447–453.

Wren TA, Rethlefsen S, Kay RM (2005) Prevalence of specific gait abnormalities in children with cerebral palsy: influence of cerebral palsy subtype, age, and previous surgery. *Journal of Pediatric Orthopaedics* **25**: 79–83.

Yaşar E, Adigüzel E, Arslan M, Matthews DJ (2018) Basics of bone metabolism and osteoporosis in common pediatric neuromuscular disabilities. *European Journal of Paediatric Neurology* **22**: 17–26.

Ôunpuu S, Deluca P, Davis R, Romness M (2002) Long-term effects of femoral derotation osteotomies: an evaluation using three-dimensional gait analysis. *Journal of Pediatric Orthopaedics* **22**: 139–145.

Accuracy in the Operating Room
A Dialogue Between a Biomedical Engineer and an Orthopaedic Surgeon

Morgan Sangeux and Thomas Dreher

KEY POINTS

- Orthopaedic surgeons involved in the care of children with cerebral palsy (CP) need to master a wide range of procedures, including muscle lengthening, tendon transfer, and bony surgeries.
- Orthopaedic surgeons and biomedical engineers routinely work together within the context of gait analysis.
- Orthopaedic surgeries in CP are mostly evaluated through pre- and post-surgery gait analyses.

OPPORTUNITIES

- Surgical navigation technologies may provide an opportunity to better control and guide orthopaedic surgeries in children with CP.
- Personalized musculoskeletal modelling provides improved estimates of muscle forces and joint contact forces during gait.

Hospital-based gait analysis laboratories generally have a team of orthopaedic surgeons, biomedical engineers or clinical scientists, and physiotherapists (Baker 2013). In this setting, the engineers are responsible for the continuous and smooth operation of the laboratory, including the collection and processing of high-quality video, motion capture, and force plate data, sometimes with the addition of electromyography and oxygen consumption data. Regular assessment of the quality and accuracy of the data produced follows written protocols and is the object of much research (McGinley et al. 2009). Gait data are then interpreted by a multidisciplinary team, including the physiotherapists and orthopaedic surgeons, in order to establish the surgical management plan.

Multidisciplinarity stops there, and rightfully so. Only the orthopaedic surgeons carry out the planned interventions. We decided to present this chapter as a dialogue between two professions that are used to working together, except, in most cases, when it comes to performing the intervention. We thought that the cross-fertilization of ideas between surgeons and engineers may be beneficial to the theme of accuracy in the operating theatre.

However, it is important to understand the difficulty and complexity of the work performed by surgeons in the operating theatre first, before one may contribute useful ideas. The following interview was conducted by a biomedical engineer, with the aim of getting a better understanding of: (1) what the overall working environment for the surgeon is like, (2) the current state of the art surgical interventions, (3) commonly faced difficulties or uncertainties, and (4) what research may be performed in the future to improve the orthopaedic care of children with cerebral palsy (CP). We tried to cover a broad range of topics, with an emphasis on bony surgery and derotation osteotomies.

SURGERIES FOR THE MANAGEMENT OF GAIT PROBLEMS IN CHILDREN WITH CP

[Morgan – Biomedical engineer]
Dear Thomas Dreher,

Thank you very much for agreeing to discuss your experience as an orthopaedic surgeon specializing in the management of children with CP.

I understand you specialize in complex surgery for children with CP. However, I wonder how much of your practice is dedicated to the management of these children and how much you also attend to more common orthopaedic problems, such as trauma?

[Thomas – Orthopaedic surgeon]
Dear Morgan Sangeux,

Thank you very much for this opportunity to discuss. It is true, my focus is on the management of complex deformities and gait disorders, and this includes neurogenic and non-neurogenic conditions. Trauma plays only a minor role, but posttraumatic deformities are common problems I deal with besides neurogenic, congenital, and idiopathic deformities.

CHANGES IN TREATMENT PHILOSOPHIES

[Morgan – Biomedical engineer]
I am interested in the type of surgery you perform to maintain or improve the capacity of children with CP to walk. I have conducted a small literature review to get an idea of the approximate proportion of surgeries performed in children with CP.

I used a recent systematic review and meta-analysis centred on multilevel surgery for children with CP (Amirmudin et al. 2019) and a few other recent studies (Dreher et al. 2018; Boyer et al. 2018; Rajagopal et al. 2018). From these, I found a wide range of results, from as low as 0% to as much as 95% for bony surgery. Muscle lengthening seems to be more predominant with a minimum of 25% and often up to 100%, while tendon transfer, release, or lengthening is performed 15% to 30% of the time. These data points are for the lower limbs only and exclude botulinum neurotoxin A injections.

Do you agree with these figures?

[Thomas – Orthopaedic surgeon]
I fully agree that there is a wide range and amount of bony and soft-tissue procedures between different publications and centres. Lack of standardization is a major problem in CP; however, due to heterogeneity

of CP, major differences in treatment philosophies, and different cultural backgrounds, the creation of a consensus is a 'mission impossible'.

Some 'leading centres' seem to develop similar approaches for the various treatments. While soft-tissue lengthening surgeries were initially done in most patients with CP, these are now less frequent, and bony surgeries to correct lever-arm dysfunctions and sparing the muscles now seem to be preferred in many centres (Dreher et al. 2018).

However, the heterogeneity of the underlying biomechanical problems requires clear and detailed analysis, and it is crucial to have both bony and soft-tissue surgeries available if indicated. It is not correct to make absolute statements for all patients.

THE RELATIONSHIP BETWEEN VOLUME AND ACCURACY

[Morgan – Biomedical engineer]

I have two questions about your experience of the difficulty to achieve technical mastery for such a wide range of procedures.

1. The relationship between surgeon volume and outcomes has been under increasing interest (Li et al. 2018; Wu et al. 2018). In total knee arthroplasty, a systematic review has shown that there was some positive relationship between the surgeon volume and the patient-reported outcomes (Lau et al. 2012), although the authors emphasized that the results should be interpreted with caution. Do you think you perform each of the surgeries children with CP need often enough to be proficient at them?

2. And, as a follow-up question, do you think it would be advisable and/or feasible for surgeons in your field to specialize in a smaller set of surgeries to finetune their performance? That is, for example, some surgeons would be specialized in derotation osteotomy, others in tendon transfer or muscle lengthening, and others in more specialized areas such as the foot or spine.

[Thomas – Orthopaedic surgeon]

1. This is a very important point. Paediatric orthopaedics cover a wide field of treatment options and especially surgical procedures. Surgeries in CP include hundreds of different techniques published at different levels, joints, muscles, and bones. Another important point is that not all centres treat the same volume of patients with CP. This clearly means that there are a lot of surgeries performed by surgeons who do not have enough volume of these specific surgeries to provide the needed routine and safety for the patient. The crucial question in this context is – what is the minimum annual number of a specific surgical procedure that qualifies a surgeon as an expert able to provide enough safety for the patient and the outcome?

   There are two things which are probably even more relevant for outcomes, and we should also discuss those. The first point is about indication. The best-skilled surgeon can perform a surgery perfectly with a bad outcome if the indication was not good. And this is something which is crucial in CP. Especially in CP, we do not have standardized indications as we have for hip osteoarthritis. Even for a 'simple' condition like hip osteoarthritis, indication for surgical treatment can be challenging.

   The other point, which is crucial, concerns the amount of intraoperative control of correction of your surgical procedure. The surgeon, as well as the indication, may be perfect, but the surgery may result in a bad outcome when intraoperative control is not sufficient.

   These two points, from my perspective, are much more crucial than the absolute experience of the surgeon and the number of patients she or he treats. Furthermore, in case more precision could be provided intraoperatively, the experience of the surgeon may not be of the highest priority to achieve the intended outcome (Stiehler et al. 2015; Wilson et al. 2016). Having said that, it is also true that the surgeon's level of experience may still play a role, even when it is supplemented with surgical navigation tools to improve precision (Lee et al. 2019).

2. It is true that it would be favourable to have a specialist for each surgical procedure, for example, during a multilevel surgery. In many adult orthopaedic hospitals, surgeons are often joint-specific specialists and are therefore focused on a limited subset of procedures and surgical approaches. However, this is difficult for paediatric orthopaedics and especially for the field of CP because a multilevel understanding of pathologies is needed and there is also a simple workforce problem.

In an 'ideal world scenario', a multilevel surgery is performed by at least six surgeons, one CP hip specialist on each side, one CP knee specialist on each side, and one CP foot and ankle specialist on each side. Procedures are performed stepwise, and the specialists assist each other during the procedures. The indication for the surgery and every single step, as well as the amount of intraoperative dosage, is determined in an interdisciplinary planning session before the surgery.

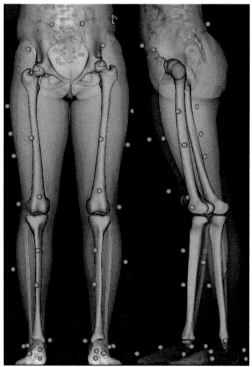

Biplane x-ray images with 3D models of the bones and markers of the lower limb superimposed (EOS imaging)

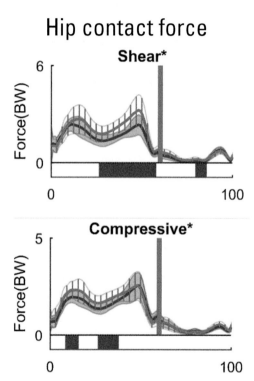

The hip joint contact forces were expressed in an acetabular coordinate system. The norm of the force in the plane of the acetabulum was labelled 'shear', and the norm of the force perpendicular to the plane was labelled 'compressive'. The red curves show the contact force for the torsioned femur and tibia while the blue curves show the contact force for normal femur and tibia torsion.

Figure 2.1 Musculoskeletal modelling and gait analysis allow us to estimate the increase in hip contact force due to torsional deformities. Simultaneous personalized skeletal geometry of the patients and registration with the motion capture markers were obtained using bi-plane x-ray imaging (EOS imaging). Adapted from Passmore et al. 2018 with permission from Elsevier.

COMMON FEMORAL AND TIBIAL BONY CORRECTIONS IN CP

[Morgan – Biomedical engineer]
I now would like to focus on bony surgery for the femur and tibia. I am aware of four main surgeries: derotation of the femur, varus and derotation of the femur, extension of the femur, and derotation of the tibia. My understanding is that the decision to perform these surgeries is mainly based on gait function, as assessed by a 3D gait analysis, rather than deviation from what is considered normal anatomy.
1. Is that the case?

2. And, once the decision is made, how do you consider anatomy and function when you plan for a certain amount of correction?

[Thomas – Orthopaedic surgeon]
1. There are many more osteotomies which may be necessary, but you are right that those four are the most common procedures and clearly need to be discussed. The decision to perform these procedures is a combination of findings during functional and anatomical evaluation (i.e. instrumented 3D gait analysis, clinical examination, and radiographic findings) (Niklasch et al. 2015b). In CP, I agree that the functional findings (gait function) are much more relevant for the decision, however, some key features from clinical examination and radiographic examinations are also essential to the decision. One example is distal femoral extension osteotomy: gait evaluation may show increased knee flexion, but in case there is no knee flexion contracture in clinical examination, extension osteotomy is not indicated.

   One major issue with the recent literature and studies is that detailed information about indications for surgical procedures is either only insufficiently reported or not reported at all. This makes the comparison and interpretation of results nearly impossible.

2. This is a difficult question and must be answered for each osteotomy separately. In principle, for rotational correction, the dynamic amount of rotational abnormality is the primary parameter which determines the amount of correction at our centre, while anatomical parameters are taken into account only secondarily, for example, to avoid unfavourable anatomical positions like femoral retroversion when correcting internal rotation or severe femoral anteversion when correcting external rotation gait. This is in accordance with the results of several publications showing overcorrection after pure anteversion correction and persistence of pelvic asymmetry, especially in asymmetrical cases (Carty et al. 2014; Schwartz et al. 2014; Niklasch et al. 2015a; Niklasch et al. 2015b). However, in many centres, indication for femoral rotation osteotomy is done according to the measurements of increased femoral anteversion associated with internal rotation gait.

   For dosage of tibia rotational osteotomy, functional and anatomical parameters (tibial torsion) are used to determine the amount of correction. Typically, tibial torsion is corrected to anatomical reference values. Intraoperative control for correction is difficult since assessment of tibial torsion intraoperatively is difficult and varies largely because of rotation in the knee and ankle joint. Some centres perform rotational correction with the patient being in prone position to be more precise in intraoperative clinical examination.

   In selected cases, tibial torsion must be corrected more or less than reference values in order to correct functional parameters.

   For sagittal plane correction (mostly extension osteotomies), intraoperative dosage of correction corresponds to the amount of knee flexion contracture, which is measured pre- and intraoperatively by clinical examination (Stout et al 2008). Functional parameters are only used to indicate this procedure but typically do not determine the amount of correction.

Frontal plane correction amounts to date are mainly determined by radiographic parameters independent of whether the correction is done at the proximal or distal femur or the proximal or distal tibia.

Clinical examination and radiographic evaluations during surgery to control for the correction amount are possible. However, it is challenging to control both rotational corrections and muscle surgeries. Since the intraoperative correction amount does not reflect functional and static outcomes, there is a need to better evaluate the effects that influence correction (Kay et al. 2000; Dreher et al. 2007).

CLINICAL RELEVANCE OF PRECISION IN ROTATIONAL CORRECTION

[Morgan – Biomedical engineer]

I was involved in research utilizing musculoskeletal modelling to investigate the effect of increased femur torsion on joint contact forces. We found that increased torsion led to increased muscle activation and forces leading to increasing hip and knee joint contact forces in children with idiopathic torsional deformities (Passmore et al. 2018), see Figure 2.1. Intuitively, one may consider that increased joint contact forces during walking is a problem for long-term joint health (Guilak 2011). However, evidence for the relationship between lower limb torsional deformities and long-term joint health is scarce and with mixed findings (Goutallier et al. 2006; Baker-LePain and Lane 2012; Li et al. 2014; Weinberg et al. 2017).

When you aim to correct bony torsion deformities, how precise do you think these need to be, and how do you control for the correction performed?

[Thomas – Orthopaedic surgeon]

The first part of your question focusses on the clinical relevance of precision of rotational correction. For sure, to date, it is difficult to prove that 1 to 4 degrees or 5 to 7 degrees or even more than this are clinically relevant for the overall correction. However, from various publications we know that the amount of intraoperative correction is only partially reflected by functional (gait analysis) and static (clinical examination, radiographic outcome) outcomes (Kay et al. 2003; Braatz et al. 2013). Furthermore, there are cases in which significant over- or under-correction occurs when evaluating individual cases. Intraoperative control for dosage may be taken into account as one major factor playing an important role in such mal-corrections. Hence, the need for precise control of what we do in the operating theatre is mandatory. On the other hand, we have to ask ourselves whether we need precise surgical planning when we are not able to provide this precision to the patient intraoperatively.

There are several options to control for rotational correction intraoperatively. Some surgeons, however, do not control it at all. A common approach to control for rotational correction is to perform the rotational correction in prone position and to use intraoperative trochanteric prominence angle test (TPAT) to determine femoral anteversion. By preoperative calculation of anteversion, the correction amount can then be derived from the difference of the preoperative anteversion and the intraoperatively measured anteversion (Davids et al. 2002).

Another common method is to use derotational K-wires, which are placed proximal and distal to the osteotomy line (Dreher et al. 2012), see Figure 2.2. These wires may be placed parallel to each other initially, and the correction in the transversal plane can then be measured after the rotational correction. Alternatively, the wires are placed in a specific rotational angle initially, and after the correction, the wires end up parallel to each other.

A further option is to mark rotation with a longitudinal line indicated with a chisel or a marker over the osteotomy and horizontally to the osteotomy line. After rotation, the amount of rotation can be calculated by measuring the distance between the two parts of the initially drawn line. The bone diameter and circumference calculations are needed for a precise calculation of the rotational amount.

Most of the existing studies to investigate the effects of rotational osteotomies lack a systematic intraoperative measurement for correction amount.

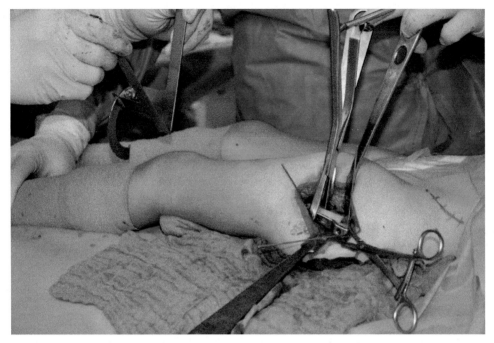

Figure 2.2 Positioning of K-wires above and below the osteotomy cut, and measurement with a goniometer.

INNOVATIVE METHODS TO IMPROVE INTRAOPERATIVE PRECISION

[Morgan – Biomedical engineer]
You recently co-authored a publication demonstrating an image-less computer-aided navigation system to measure the correction in real-time using active electromagnetic sensors (Geisbusch et al. 2017). Can you tell me more about the decision to develop such a protocol and the choices you made?

For example, you used electromagnetic technology to track instrumented K-wires while most navigation systems use optoelectronic technology. You also decided to restrict yourself with an image-less system to track the correction, rather than guide the insertion of the guide wires and blade, which may have required 3D modelling of the bones from medical imaging.

[Thomas – Orthopaedic surgeon]
For the sagittal and frontal plane, clinical examination and intraoperative imaging represent established methods to control for correction amount and over- or under-correction can be measured fairly accurately. However, the control of the transversal plane is difficult and even when derotational K-wires are used, the number of potential measurement errors is high. Furthermore, the interrater reliability of intraoperative rotational measurements is weak even in an in vitro environment using sawbone models where the K-wires can be perfectly seen and the examiner can measure from an optimum position, which is not possible in the operating room where soft-tissue does not lead to difficulties of measuring. Despite satisfactory

overall outcomes after rotational correction, there is large variability in the expected outcome of individual patients. To be more precise and eliminate the potential of intraoperative dosage errors as one major factor influencing the postoperative outcome, we searched for options to better control for rotational correction amount during surgery.

The idea was that we use the standard surgery setting for rotational control so that no additional pre-operative imaging nor additional invasive intraoperative setups are needed to measure rotation. This is one reason why we have not chosen optoelectronic technology because additional placement of reference guides is needed. Furthermore, the functionality of the camera-system depends on the positioning of the surgeons. This is not the case for the Emergency Medical Technician (EMT) system, which also allows for continuous monitoring of rotational correction during the whole surgery (Geisbusch et al. 2017), see Figure 2.3.

We initially thought rotational amount was the only parameter we needed to monitor and that the system was developed just for monitoring. However, we have learned that several steps of the surgical procedure may influence the rotational correction, including the plane of the osteotomy, the plate type, the plate fixation, and the screw fixation. We are currently working on further developing the system to be able to use it as a guiding system for the whole surgical procedure rather than just monitoring transversal plane correction.

[Morgan – Biomedical engineer]
One study showed that a computer-assisted navigation system improved accuracy for high tibial osteotomy, notably in less experienced surgeons (Takao et al. 2017). However, navigation systems may present steep learning curves that could be difficult to overcome in low volume surgeries. What is your experience of this in the system you developed?

[Thomas – Orthopaedic surgeon]
Since I have witnessed the whole process of developing the system, I can report that we have experienced a lot of limitations, which resulted in significant changes and improvements to the system itself. Meanwhile, we are at the stage that a prototype for clinical use is ready. The system itself is very simple to use, and this is a clear advantage. However, like every new system, there is a need for a thorough tutorial on how to use it and the potential sources of error. One major problem is the influence of massive steel instruments on the electromagnetic field in case they come too close to the electrodes. Furthermore, the positioning of the electromagnetic generator is a challenge because it may interfere with intraoperative radiographic imaging. Aside from these limitations, the system is easy to use and does not require much additional time and effort during the surgery. However, there are options to solve such problems.

[Morgan – Biomedical engineer]
Most research into the use of computer-assisted osteotomy is focused on high tibial osteotomy (HTO; open wedge or closed wedge) in adults. The findings in HTO highlight the increase in precision when using the navigation system, but maybe indicate a lack of translation to clinical outcomes. How would you plan the research effort in image-less navigation system for femur derotation? And what would be the outcome measures?

[Thomas – Orthopaedic surgeon]
Unfortunately, again adult treatment is more advanced than paediatric care. HTO is a perfect example where an extraordinary amount of precision is claimed by several authors. However, as you have correctly identified, the precision claimed is not yet proven to be relevant for clinical outcomes. However, long-term

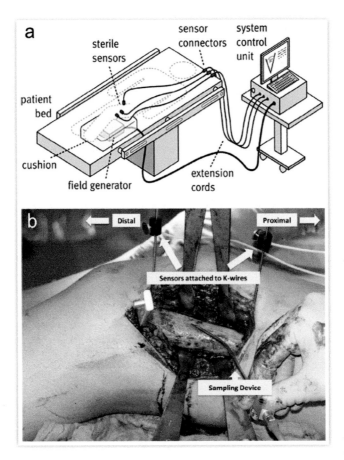

Figure 2.3 Schematic of the Emergency Medical Technician system (EMT). Reprinted from Geisbusch et al. 2017 with permission from Wiley.

studies have not proven that precision is unnecessary, and we should make sure results are as precise as possible in cases with HTO. A comparison with precision in surgeries for children with CP is not valid since HTO is done to counteract the development of osteoarthritis in the future. Rotational corrections in children with CP are not mainly done for prevention of osteoarthritis, but mainly to correct a functionally disturbing internal rotation gait.

We are running a randomized controlled trial, where half of the patients with corrective osteotomies are treated with the use of intraoperative monitoring with EMT, while the other half are treated with conventional goniometric measurements. The primary outcome parameter of this study is the change in rotation according to torsional magnetic resonance imaging or computed tomography (CT). This study aims to prove that the precision of planned correction is higher using the EMT system. This study includes 3D gait analysis before and after at specific follow-up examinations to evaluate whether the precision of using EMT for monitoring has a positive effect on gait function.

Future studies will need to focus on other planes and whether the advantages of more precision remain favourable in the long-term. The opportunity to use such systems to guide the surgical procedure is important to investigate whether impression depending on the level of experience of the surgeon can be ruled out.

[Morgan – Biomedical engineer]

My understanding is that often femur derotation is associated with a varus correction to prevent potential hip dysplasia.

In theory, this image-less navigation system could monitor correction in two planes, but in practice, 3D medical images are often required. Recently, I came across the use of a personalized 3D printed guide to assist with the blade insertion and improve the precision of the planned correction. The 3D printed guide required 3D medical imaging to design and plan the surgery but seemed to reduce both the intra-operative surgery time and intraoperative need for medical imaging (Zheng et al. 2017). What is your opinion about the strengths and weaknesses of this type of technology? And, what would be the research required to investigate further the potential of such technology in children with CP?

[Thomas – Orthopaedic surgeon]

Yes, often there is a need for 2D, 3D, or even 4D modelling (with shortening) correction osteotomy for femoral derotation. Since I started working in Zurich, I have used 3D printed guides for individualized complex deformity correction, including in cases with neurogenic conditions such as CP, see Figure 2.4.

One major advantage is that the preoperative planning and the individualized 3D prints reduce the potential sources of mal-correction intraoperatively. Furthermore, the dependence of the postoperative results on the surgeon's skills and experience is less relevant. Such systems even allow preplanning of the type and position of fixation methods (plates, screws, nails, etc.).

Disadvantages include the need for preoperative CT scans for 3D bone reconstruction, much larger surgical approaches compared to conventional surgical techniques, and limited intraoperative draw-back options in case the correction is incorrect. Furthermore, costs could be a relevant factor in everyday practice.

A relevant and major issue with such an approach for correction is that the system references anatomical reconstruction, which does not necessarily fit the function as discussed earlier. Therefore, functional data must be included in the planning of the correction and corrective 3D guides.

Research in the field of individualized 3D guides for use in patients with CP should focus on how much precision of specific corrections can be improved by using such technologies and how individualized evaluation of anatomy corresponds to functional findings during gait analysis. Furthermore, the flexibility of 3D guides according to intraoperative examination results after correction of other planes needs to be verified.

[Morgan – Biomedical engineer]

I have one more question before we leave the topic of femur derotation osteotomy. There are several techniques to guide the growth of the long bones of the lower limb in children, in order to induce progressive corrections in the coronal and sagittal planes. I came across several studies, first in rabbits (Arami et al. 2013), then in children (Metaizeau et al. 2019), that used guided growth to induce progressive rotational corrections, about 1.2 degrees per month in children aged 10 years old, (Metaizeau et al. 2019) Figure 2.5. The consequence of the rotational correction was a reduction of the longitudinal growth. These techniques may have some advantages in terms of reduced time to recover from the surgery. They may also provide an opportunity to investigate the sole effect of a decrease in torsional deformity on gait through fixed-time interval longitudinal gait analysis studies during the period of correction.

However, the techniques are recent (between 2013 and 2015) and have only been tested in a few centres. Do you think rotational guided growth may offer some insight into the relationship between torsional deformity and gait, and provide an alternative to conventional derotation osteotomy?

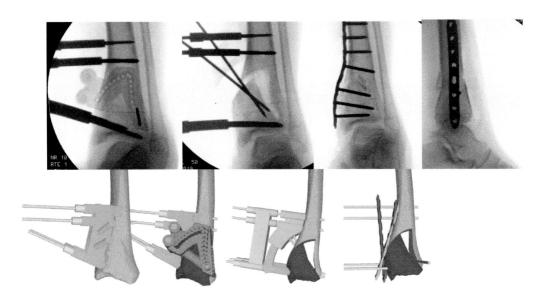

Figure 2.4 Application of a 3D printed guide to control osteotomy of the tibia.

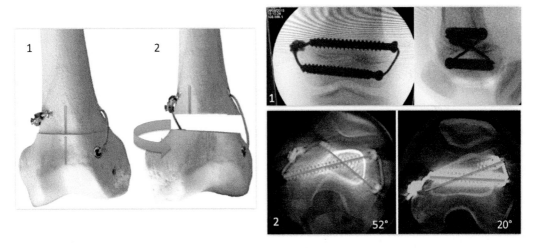

Figure 2.5 Principal of progressive rotational correction with growth in children with femur torsional deformities. Adapted from Metaizeau et al. 2019 with permission from Elsevier.

[Thomas – Orthopaedic surgeon]

The results of the cited studies show that the change of rotation is variable and dependant on the surgical technique and positioning of the implants. The cost of a reduction in longitudinal growth may also be an issue. The idea of having the opportunity to control the sagittal plane during growth in children with CP is interesting, but it seems that the approach to modify the growth plate just to correct the rotation is not ideal. As these methods are not proven to be controllable concerning timing and amount of correction, as well as adverse effects, these methods seem unsuitable for the treatment of rotational correction in CP.

However, your question got me thinking. For surgical lengthening of the tibia or femur, there is a method to implant a nail, which can be expanded by a magnetic mechanism that is typically used a few days after the nail implantation and after the bone has been osteotomized (Kirane et al. 2014). A major problem in CP is imprecise correction (over- or under-correction) or recurrence of deformities during growth. If an implant can be re-activated for adjusting the correction, which was not precise enough during the surgery or correcting the deformity again which was recurrent after several years, many problems in the treatment of associated gait problems and deformities in CP could be solved.

TIBIA CORRECTIVE OSTEOTOMIES IN CP

[Morgan – Biomedical engineer]

Let's now focus on the tibia, which is often (de)rotated as well. I am under the impression that there are fewer practical difficulties and that surgeons tend to better control the derotation of the tibia. Would you agree? Or should there be some concerted research and development efforts towards improving the precision of tibia surgery?

[Thomas – Orthopaedic surgeon]

Additional tibial rotational corrections have a relevant influence on the overall transversal alignment of the limb and should therefore not be forgotten when talking about a transversal plane correction in CP.

To focus on your questions and impressions, I find the control of derotation or rotation of the tibia more difficult than for the femur. This is because of several reasons, including the rotation between the tibia and the fibula, the rotation in the knee joint, and the difficulty of defining tibial torsion as well as foot rotation. Other colleagues state that they find tibial transversal correction easier than femoral torsional correction because the aim of tibial correction in most cases is a restoration of normal tibial torsion. However, further research is needed to:

1. Improve the detection of tibial torsion and the correlation with dynamic parameters.
2. Measure tibial torsion during gait.
3. Include the amount of tibial torsion into the treatment plan.
4. Improve control for tibial rotational correction intraoperatively.
5. Reference tibial torsion intraoperatively.

FOOT SURGERY IN CHILDREN WITH CP

[Morgan – Biomedical engineer]

Let's move further distally and talk about foot surgery. The foot lever is essential for the support of body weight and forward progression, but it is also often compromised in children with CP. It seems the foot and ankle are two of the main locations of pain, both in children (Alriksson-Schmidt and Hagglund 2016) and in adults (Opheim et al. 2011).

Are you satisfied with the precision of foot lever surgical correction or enhancement?

[Thomas – Orthopaedic surgeon]

To answer this question, we need to clarify the goals for surgical foot correction in the context of multilevel surgery in children and adolescents with CP. Typically, what we need for an optimum lever-arm function is a plantigrade foot which is able to adequately dorsiflex the ankle during loading response, have enough control of second rocker movement, have a stable and controlled passive dorsiflexion in mid- and late stance to control plantarflexion/knee extension couple, and have enough plantar- and dorsiflexion motion during the swing phase of gait (Perry 1992). During the stance phase, foot lever plays an important role in knee positioning and motion, as well as hip motion.

During surgery, lever-arm reconstruction in the foot is done with stabilizing osteotomies or arthrodesis or combinations of both (Fulford 1990; Yoo et al. 2005; Park et al. 2008; El-Hilaly et al. 2019). Stability of the foot is tested manually in the operating room, and the changes in bony architecture can be quantified using intraoperative radiographic imaging. However, I am not aware of any other published method monitoring or guiding intraoperative precision of bony foot correction.

To strive for precision in the operating room, the amount of correction needed has to be determined before the surgery, and this means detailed planning. It is an interesting question of whether we are able to clearly quantify instability and deformity by different imaging and testing before surgery and to define the desired outcome parameters to develop an algorithm for intraoperative precision control.

Specific foot models in 3D gait analysis are helpful in quantifying motion of specific foot segments during gait (Liu et al. 2014; Beckmann et al. 2015; Kruger et al. 2017; Amene et al. 2019) and provide important parameters to monitor the effects of surgical correction in foot deformities (Dreher et al. 2014). In the future, it would be desirable to also consider specific foot models for planning the surgical procedures and to determine intraoperative dosage of correction.

[Morgan – Biomedical engineer]
That's all the questions I had about bony surgeries performed in children with CP. Is there anything else you would like to mention before we move on to soft tissue surgeries?

[Thomas – Orthopaedic surgeon]
We did not talk about osteotomies for patella advancement, which is seen as a key procedure during crouch gait management. Intraoperatively, patella height is typically used as the primary parameter to check for correction amount. However, sometimes it is difficult to determine the desired amount of correction. Can you as an engineer think about methods to control for correction of patella advancement? In particular, how can we measure triceps femoris and rectus femoris tension during this procedure?

[Morgan – Biomedical engineer]
Excellent question. This is a typical case where musculoskeletal modelling may provide some insights and help with planning by providing some optimal correction targets. I am aware of the work of Bittmann et al. (Bittmann et al. 2018) (see Chapter 9) who investigated the effect of the position of the patella (alta pre-surgery/normal/baja sometimes post-surgery) on the knee extension moment-arm for various degrees of knee flexion. The study investigated the mechanical effect of the position of the patella pre- and post-surgery retrospectively, utilizing x-ray imaging.

It is important to note that only detailed documentation and pre- and post-measurements of the anatomical variables of interest allows us to conduct such musculoskeletal modelling studies. Therefore, any tool navigation systems or medical imaging aiming to improve the precision of the planned correction may also enhance the possibility to conduct such musculoskeletal modelling studies in the future.

SOFT TISSUE PROCEDURES

[Morgan – Biomedical engineer]
My understanding of most muscle lengthening procedures is that the muscle aponeurosis, or its tendon in extreme cases, is damaged somehow, and the lengthening occurs by acting on the adjacent joint to increase its range of movement, which pulls on (tear) and lengthens the muscle. Is this a reasonable summary?

[Thomas – Orthopaedic surgeon]

This is mostly correct. In principle, we have to distinguish three types of muscle-tendon techniques for lengthening. First, aponeurotic lengthening where the aponeurosis of a muscle is cut, typically horizontally, and the underlying muscle is spared. The incision can be done on one or more levels in order to control for the amount of correction. By stretching the muscle, lengthening of the muscle-tendon unit is achieved. Another option is to lengthen the tendon itself at a point where no muscle tissue is present anymore. Z- or U-shaped cuts of the tendon lead to a lengthening effect, and the tendon is sutured after the desired length is achieved. Lastly, tenotomy can be performed where the tendon is purely cut allowing a joint better passive range of motion but at the cost of lost function of the muscle of which the tendon was cut.

[Morgan – Biomedical engineer]

Do you systematically measure, for example, using a goniometer or any other intraoperative instrumented measurement tools (e.g. instrumented measure for passive ankle dorsiflexion [Hastings-Ison et al. 2014]), the initial and final range of movement of the joint?

[Thomas – Orthopaedic surgeon]

Yes, we use a special goniometer in the operating room to measure, for example, the popliteal angle and the modified popliteal angle before and after lengthening procedure. We use the same technique for the intraoperative Silfverskiöld test.

[Morgan – Biomedical engineer]

What do we know about the effect of the lengthening procedure on the overall muscle? It seems, to me, that the procedure operates on the superficial layer of the muscle (when it is performed to the aponeurosis), and it is not clear, to me, how the superficial lengthening translates to the deeper muscle tissue. Are you aware of any studies that investigated the effect of the procedure on increasing tissue depth on the fascicles and/or even the fibres?

Also, how does the tissue remodel from the procedure?

[Thomas – Orthopaedic surgeon]

No, there is definitely a need for more investigation.

[Morgan – Biomedical engineer]

In the case of a muscle release, i.e. the complete section of the muscle-tendon, as I believe is performed to the adductors, do you have any means to measure the length of the muscle retraction?

And, have you experienced large variability of retraction length in patients?

[Thomas – Orthopaedic surgeon]

There are different techniques for lengthening the adductors. In principle, I do not recommend tenotomy of the adductors in ambulatory children with CP, I prefer fractional intramuscular lengthening.

Concerning your question about measuring the retraction, there is currently no measuring technique, and I believe that in cases where we perform tenotomies measuring the amount of retraction is clinically of minor relevance. However, it is of great interest to measure the amount of retraction during fractional intramuscular lengthening or during tendon Z-lengthening and put this into relation with the amount of achieved correction. This could represent an important tool for controlling the intraoperative dosage of such a procedure. Dynamic muscle length during walking could also be an important parameter for the determination on how much length we have to gain by a surgical lengthening procedure.

Another important topic is how much tension do we need when we reconstruct the tendon after a lengthening. Currently there is no helpful data available.

[Morgan – Biomedical engineer]
The last topic I have for us to discuss is tendon transfer surgery. We know that simulations using musculoskeletal models are the most sensitive to a parameter called slack length, the length at which the muscle-tendon unit starts to produce passive tension (Ackland et al. 2012). Therefore, it is likely the tension at which the tendon is re-attached after the transfer would have a large effect on function. How do you control the tension?

And, have you had cases where you attributed later problems during the patient rehabilitation to a too low or too high re-attachment tension during surgery?

[Thomas – Orthopaedic surgeon]
There is no systematic way of controlling the tension after transfer or lengthening. Typically, I fix the transfer by pulling the transferred tendon with a 'medium' tension, but this term is flawed and significantly depends on the person who is pulling the tendon. A more standardized approach to control for this 'tension' and the associated resulting effects on the overall muscle-tendon length as well as on muscle velocity during walking would be desirable.

I have had cases where the tension in the tendon after re-attachment was probably too high or too low, as I am sure most surgeons performing these surgeries have experienced. If there is a way to better control it and to clearly define for the individual patient how much tension is necessary, I believe that we could avoid or at least limit the number of over- or under-corrected cases.

CONCLUSION

The need for additional tools to better control the amount of correction performed during surgery has been mentioned several times in this interview. Orthopaedic surgeons specializing in the care of children with CP need to be both one-person bands, able to perform a wide range of surgeries, and virtuoso performers highly skilled in each of the surgeries performed. In this context, there is a need for tools to measure the key parameter(s) the surgeon aims to adjust with surgery in real-time and with proper feedback.

Surgical navigation systems have improved the precision of total knee or hip joint arthroplasty and improve accuracy in high tibial wedge osteotomies (Hasan et al. 2015). The EMT system presented above is the first attempt to bring the benefits of surgical navigation to the derotation osteotomy of the femur. Personalized 3D printed guides may be another solution to improve control, especially when surgical correction needs to occur in several planes (Zheng et al. 2017).

Tools to measure and control the number of soft tissue surgeries focus on the effect on the range of movement at the joint of interest. However, it seems that little is known about the effect on the structure of the soft tissue itself. For example, what is the exact intramuscular amount of lengthening/stretching, and how does the lengthening propagate within the depth of the muscle? For tendon transfer, the key parameter of the tension at which the tendon is re-attached is not measured. Some solutions exist and have been experimented on in other areas of surgery. For example, tensioning devices have been used to control tendon tension during rotator cuff repair surgery (Park et al. 2019) or to measure the tension of an anterior cruciate ligament graft (Nishizawa et al. 2017). Ultrasound imaging, coupled with a tapping mechanical stimulus, may also be used to measure force in vivo and non-invasively (Martin et al. 2018). Further research and developments towards feasible and safe measurement of soft tissue surgery performed in children with CP seems warranted.

Finally, the question of how precise surgery needs to be is a difficult one to answer. First and foremost, the relationship between structure (e.g. femur torsion) and function (e.g. during gait) is not straightforward in children with CP. Surgeons, and the multidisciplinary team supporting them, require time and experience to acquire judgment mastery. Musculoskeletal modelling may be used to explore the effect of a range of parameters that may be corrected through surgery (bone shape or position, tendon tension, muscle lengthening) on muscle forces and joint contact forces during gait and other activities. However, the relationship between these biomechanical variables and clinical outcomes or patient satisfaction is not straightforward either. The relationship between biomechanical variables and long-term clinical consequences, for example, the effect of repetitive increased hip joint contact forces on acetabulum cartilage health is, therefore, another area where further research seems warranted.

5-YEAR PRIORITIES

- **Document procedures:** Keep precise records of the type, location, and surgical techniques for all procedures performed.
- **Measure procedures:** Record and report the actual size of the correction performed, e.g. femur derotation of 10 degrees, using precise measurement instruments. Pre- and post-medical imaging and navigation systems may be useful for that.
- **Further develop navigation systems and 3D printed guide for surgeries in multiple planes.**
- **Investigate effects of progressive correction:** Longitudinal gait analysis assessments during progressive derotation during growth may improve our understanding of the effect of torsional deformities on gait.

FUTURE NEEDS

- **Translating model outputs to clinical effects:** Musculoskeletal models now better estimate muscle and joint contact forces during gait, but investigations are required to understand how these altered forces translate to clinical consequences.

REFERENCES

Ackland DC, Lin YC, Pandy MG (2012) Sensitivity of model predictions of muscle function to changes in moment arms and muscle-tendon properties: a Monte-Carlo analysis. *J Biomech* **45**: 1463–1471.

Alriksson-Schmidt A, Hagglund G (2016) Pain in children and adolescents with cerebral palsy: a population-based registry study. *Acta Paediatr* **105**: 665–670.

Amene J, Krzak JJ, Kruger KM et al. (2019) Kinematic foot types in youth with pes planovalgus secondary to cerebral palsy. *Gait Posture* **68**: 430-436.

Amirmudin NA, Lavelle G, Theologis T, Thompson N, Ryan JM (2019) Multilevel Surgery for Children With Cerebral Palsy: A Meta-analysis. *Pediatrics* **143**.

Arami A, Bar-On E, Herman A, Velkes S, Heller S (2013) Guiding femoral rotational growth in an animal model. *J Bone Joint Surg Am* **95**: 2022–2027.

Baker-Lepain JC, Lane NE (2012) Role of bone architecture and anatomy in osteoarthritis. *Bone* **51**: 197–203.

Baker R (2013) *Measuring Walking: A Handbook of Clinical Gait Analysis*. Cambridge: Mac Keith Press.

Beckmann NA, Wolf SI, Heitzmann D, Wallroth A, Muller S, Dreher T (2015) Cavovarus deformity in Charcot-Marie-Tooth disease: is there a hindfoot equinus deformity that needs treatment? *J Foot Ankle Res* **8**: 65.

Bittmann MF, Lenhart RL, Schwartz MH, Novacheck TF, Hetzel S, Thelen DG (2018) How does patellar tendon advancement alter the knee extensor mechanism in children treated for crouch gait? *Gait Posture* **64**: 248–254.

Boyer ER, Stout JL, Laine JC et al. (2018) Long-Term Outcomes of Distal Femoral Extension Osteotomy and Patellar Tendon Advancement in Individuals with Cerebral Palsy. *J Bone Joint Surg Am* **100**: 31–41.

Braatz F, Wolf SI, Gerber A, Klotz MC, Dreher T (2013) Do changes in torsional magnetic resonance imaging reflect improvement in gait after femoral derotation osteotomy in patients with cerebral palsy? *Int Orthop* **37**: 2193–2198.

Carty CP, Walsh HP, Gillett JG et al. (2014) The effect of femoral derotation osteotomy on transverse plane hip and pelvic kinematics in children with cerebral palsy: a systematic review and meta-analysis. *Gait Posture* **40**: 333–340.

Davids JR, Benfanti P, Blackhurst DW, Allen BL (2002) Assessment of femoral anteversion in children with cerebral palsy: Accuracy of the trochanteric prominence angle test. *Journal of Pediatric Orthopaedics* **22**: 173–178.

Dreher T, Thomason P, Svehlik M et al. (2018) Long-term development of gait after multilevel surgery in children with cerebral palsy: a multicentre cohort study. *Dev Med Child Neurol* **60**: 88–93.

Dreher T, Wolf S, Braatz F, Patikas D, Döderlein L (2007) Internal rotation gait in spastic diplegia-Critical considerations for the femoral derotation osteotomy. *Gait and Posture* **26**: 25–31.

Dreher T, Wolf SI, Heitzmann D, Fremd C, Klotz MC, Wenz W (2014) Tibialis posterior tendon transfer corrects the foot drop component of cavovarus foot deformity in Charcot-Marie-Tooth disease. *J Bone Joint Surg Am* **96**: 456–462.

Dreher T, Wolf SI, Heitzmann D et al. (2012) Long-term outcome of femoral derotation osteotomy in children with spastic diplegia. *Gait Posture* **36**: 467–470.

El-Hilaly R, El-Sherbini MH, Abd-Ella MM, Omran AA (2019) Radiological outcome of calcaneo-cuboid-cuneiform osteotomies for planovalgus feet in cerebral palsy children: Relationship with pedobarography. *Foot Ankle Surg* **25**: 462–468.

Fulford GE (1990 Surgical management of ankle and foot deformities in cerebral palsy. *Clin Orthop Relat Res* 55–61.

Geisbusch A, Auer C, Dickhaus H, Putz C, Dreher T (2017) Electromagnetic tracking for femoral derotation osteotomy-an in vivo study. *J Orthop Res* **35**: 2652–2657.

Goutallier D, Van Driessche S, Manicom O, Sariali E, Bernageau J, Radier C (2006) Influence of lower-limb torsion on long-term outcomes of tibial valgus osteotomy for medial compartment knee osteoarthritis. *J Bone Joint Surg Am* **88**: 2439–2447.

Guilak F (2011) Biomechanical factors in osteoarthritis. *Best Pract Res Clin Rheumatol* **25**: 815–823.

Hasan K, Rahman QA, Zalzal P (2015) Navigation versus conventional high tibial osteotomy: systematic review. *Springerplus* 4: 271.

Hastings-Ison T, Blackburn C, Opie NL et al. (2014) Reproducibility of an instrumented measure for passive ankle dorsiflexion in conscious and anaesthetized children with cerebral palsy. *Dev Med Child Neurol* **56**: 378–385.

Kay RM, Dennis S, Rethlefsen S, Reynolds RA, Skaggs DL, Tolo VT (2000) The effect of preoperative gait analysis on orthopaedic decision making. *Clin Orthop Relat Res* **372**: 217–222.

Kay RM, Rethlefsen SA, Hale JM, Skaggs DL, Tolo VT (2003) Comparison of proximal and distal rotational femoral osteotomy in children with cerebral palsy. *J Pediatr Orthop* **23**: 150–154.

Kirane YM, Fragomen AT, Rozbruch SR (2014) Precision of the PRECICE internal bone lengthening nail. *Clin Orthop Relat Res* **472**: 3869–3878.

Kruger KM, Konop KA, Krzak JJ et al. (2017) Segmental kinematic analysis of planovalgus feet during walking in children with cerebral palsy. *Gait Posture* **54**: 277–283.

Lau RL, Perruccio AV, Gandhi R, Mahomed NN (2012) The role of surgeon volume on patient outcome in total knee arthroplasty: a systematic review of the literature. *BMC Musculoskelet Disord* **13**: 250.

Lee HW, Song SJ, Bae DK, Park CH (2019) The influence of computer-assisted surgery experience on the accuracy and precision of the postoperative mechanical axis during computer-assisted lateral closing-wedge high tibial osteotomy. *Knee Surgery & Related Research* **31**: 15.

Li H, Wang Y, Oni JK et al. (2014) The role of femoral neck anteversion in the development of osteoarthritis in dysplastic hips. *Bone Joint J* **96**: 1586–1593.

Li HZ, Lin Z, Li ZZ et al. (2018) Relationship between surgeon volume and outcomes in spine surgery: a dose-response meta-analysis. *Ann Transl Med* **6**: 441.

Liu XC, Embrey D, Tassone C et al. (2014) Foot and ankle joint movements inside orthoses for children with spastic CP. *J Orthop Res* **32**: 531–536.

Martin JA, Brandon SCE, Keuler EM et al. (2018) Gauging force by tapping tendons. *Nat Commun* **9**: 1592.

Mcginley JL, Baker R, Wolfe R, Morris ME (2009) The reliability of three-dimensional kinematic gait measurements: a systematic review. *Gait Posture* **29**: 360–369.

Metaizeau JD, Denis D, Louis D (2019) New femoral derotation technique based on guided growth in children. *Orthop Traumatol Surg Res* **105**: 1175–1179.

Niklasch M, Doderlein L, Klotz MC, Braatz F, Wolf SI, Dreher T (2015a) Asymmetric pelvic and hip rotation in children with bilateral cerebral palsy: uni- or bilateral femoral derotation osteotomy? *Gait Posture* **41**: 670–675.

Niklasch M, Dreher T, Doderlein L et al. (2015b) Superior functional outcome after femoral derotation osteotomy according to gait analysis in cerebral palsy. *Gait Posture* **41**: 52–56.

Nishizawa Y, Hoshino Y, Nagamune K et al. (2017) Comparison Between Intra- and Extra-articular Tension of the Graft During Fixation in Anterior Cruciate Ligament Reconstruction. *Arthroscopy* **33**: 1204–1210.

Opheim A, Jahnsen R, Olsson E, Stanghelle JK (2011) Physical and mental components of health-related quality of life and musculoskeletal pain sites over seven years in adults with spastic cerebral palsy. *J Rehabil Med* **43**: 382–387.

Park KB, Park HW, Lee KS, Joo SY, Kim HW (2008) Changes in dynamic foot pressure after surgical treatment of valgus deformity of the hindfoot in cerebral palsy. *J Bone Joint Surg Am* **90**: 1712–1721.

Park SG, Shim BJ, Seok HG (2019) How Much Will High Tension Adversely Affect Rotator Cuff Repair Integrity? *Arthroscopy* **35**: 2992–3000.

Passmore E, Graham HK, Pandy MG, Sangeux M (2018) Hip- and patellofemoral-joint loading during gait are increased in children with idiopathic torsional deformities. *Gait Posture* **63**: 228–235.

Perry J (1992) *Gait Analysis Normal and Pathological Function.* New Jersey: SLACK Incorporated.

Rajagopal A, Kidzinski L, Mcglaughlin AS, Hicks JL, Delp SL, Schwartz MH (2018) Estimating the effect size of surgery to improve walking in children with cerebral palsy from retrospective observational clinical data. *Sci Rep* **8**: 16344.

Schwartz MH, Rozumalski A, Novacheck TF (2014) Femoral derotational osteotomy: surgical indications and outcomes in children with cerebral palsy. *Gait Posture* **39**: 778–783.

Stiehler M, Goronzy J, Kirschner S, Hartmann A, Schafer T, Gunther KP (2015) Effect of surgical experience on imageless computer-assisted femoral component positioning in hip resurfacing – a preclinical study. *Eur J Med Res* **20**: 18.

Stout JL, Gage JR, Schwartz MH, Novacheck TF (2008) Distal femoral extension osteotomy and patellar tendon advancement to treat persistent crouch gait in cerebral palsy. *J Bone Joint Surg Am* **90**: 2470–2484.

Takao M, Nishii T, Sakai T, Sugano N (2017) Comparison of rotational acetabular osteotomy performed with navigation by surgeons with different levels of experience of osteotomies. *Int J Comput Assist Radiol Surg* **12**: 841–853.

Weinberg DS, Park PJ, Morris WZ, Liu RW (2017) Femoral Version and Tibial Torsion are Not Associated With Hip or Knee Arthritis in a Large Osteological Collection. *J Pediatr Orthop* **37**: e120–e128.

Wilson MD, Dowsey MM, Spelman T, Choong PF (2016) Impact of surgical experience on outcomes in total joint arthroplasties. *ANZ J Surg* **86**: 967–972.

Wu XD, Liu MM, Sun YY et al. (2018) Relationship between hospital or surgeon volume and outcomes in joint arthroplasty: protocol for a suite of systematic reviews and dose-response meta-analyses. *BMJ Open* **8**: e022797.

Yoo WJ, Chung CY, Choi IH, Cho TJ, Kim DH (2005) Calcaneal lengthening for the planovalgus foot deformity in children with cerebral palsy. *J Pediatr Orthop* **25**: 781–785.

Zheng P, Xu P, Yao Q, Tang K, Lou Y (2017) 3D-printed navigation template in proximal femoral osteotomy for older children with developmental dysplasia of the hip. *Sci Rep* **7**: 44993.

Outcome Measurement in Ambulatory Cerebral Palsy

Benjamin J Shore, Kaat Desloovere, and Unni G Narayanan

KEY POINTS

- Clinicians must evaluate the effectiveness of their interventions and management strategies.
- Outcome measures must be reliable, valid, and sensitive to change.
- Different stakeholders have different perspectives about the importance of different outcomes.
- No single measure covers all domains of importance; a range of measures may be required to assess a child with ambulatory cerebral palsy (CP) comprehensively.
- The effectiveness of an intervention should be judged using meaningful patient-reported outcome measures that reflect the goals and expectations of patients and their parents.
- Patient-specific technical outcomes can inform patient and parent goals and be monitored longitudinally for treatment planning, evaluation of treatment algorithms, and to evaluate effectiveness of interventions from a technical perspective.

OPPORTUNITIES AND FUTURE DIRECTIONS

- Portable technology may expand the area of gait data capture in the real world.
- Utilization of computer adaptive testing platforms may enhance our ability to capture outcomes on our patients more efficiently.
- Goal based patient reported outcome measures (PROMs) might facilitate shared decision making as well as outcome assessment.
- Development of international, multi-center registries and databases that capture common data elements and outcome measures longitudinally will facilitate more robust methods for analysis of multiple variables including Artificial Intelligence.
- Databases of standardized outcome parameters may serve as input for treatment prediction algorithms.

Ambulatory children with cerebral palsy (CP) are subjected to a multitude of interventions throughout childhood to preserve or improve their gait-related function. These interventions include various forms of physical therapy, orthoses, local or systemic management of hypertonia by medical or neurosurgical procedures, and orthopedic surgery. There is wide variation in the application of these potentially complementary and competing strategies. There is an imperative to establish whether these interventions make a meaningful difference to the lives of these children and whether these benefits last into adulthood. This chapter reviews current concepts of outcome measurement, highlighting frameworks for the conceptualization of outcomes, and discussing the role of both technical and patient/parent-reported outcomes that are pertinent to ambulatory children with CP.

Case Scenario

Let's consider a typical patient with ambulatory CP. Alex is an 11-year old male with bilateral spastic CP who walks with a jump gait pattern. He walks on tiptoes with his knees flexed. His feet and his knees are turned inward. His knees rub against each other and, he trips frequently. He is less tolerant of his ankle-foot orthoses (AFOs), which cause his feet to blister and hurt. He tires easily and finds it difficult to keep up with his friends. He is relying more on a walker even for shorter distances. On examination, he has equinus contractures arising primarily from the gastrocnemius, contractures of the hamstrings without knee flexion contractures, and excessive femoral anteversion. Following 3D gait analysis, he undergoes multilevel orthopedic surgery to improve his gait. Six months after surgery and extensive physiotherapy, he walks with his heels down and his feet pointing straight. His knees come to full extension during stance and no longer rub against each other. He uses a walker at home and school and a wheelchair in the community. He is tolerant of his AFOs. He experiences hypersensitivity in his feet and finds it difficult to take steps in his bare feet. His walking speed and endurance declined in the first few months after surgery but have recently improved but not exceeded his preoperative level. Has the intervention made Alex better? How can we measure this?

WHAT ARE OUTCOMES?

Outcomes are the consequences of an intervention or what happens over time (natural history) without treatment (Natsch et al. 2003). An intervention is effective when it alters the natural history of that condition favorably and achieves its goals. When an intervention is prescribed to address a symptom or problem, the treatment goals are reactive. For our patient Alex, some of the reactive goals include addressing his tripping, foot pain and blistering, and his fatigue. Goals are preventive or prophylactic when the treatment is prescribed to prevent or mitigate some future problems (e.g. painful osteoarthritis, loss of independent walking). In the case of Alex, who functions at a Gross Motor Function Classification System (GMFCS) level III, his functional level might deteriorate as he grows taller and heavier during adolescence. An important preventive goal would be to preserve his function.

Different outcomes can be expected to occur at different times. Some are noted early (e.g. improved gait pattern), while other outcomes occur later (e.g. improved walking speed and distance). Not all outcomes are desirable (benefits). Some outcomes can be undesirable (harms), which might be expected (e.g. postoperative pain, muscle weakness) or unexpected – complications or adverse events (e.g. dysesthesias in the feet following nerve stretch injury). These harmful outcomes can be transient or permanent. Similarly, in the context of ambulatory CP, the benefits might be short-lived (e.g. following botulinum neurotoxin A injection) or expected to last a long time. In growing children, some outcomes might be lost over time. Will the gains Alex has made following surgery be sustained as he goes through his adolescent growth spurt, or is he likely to experience recurrent contractures?

FRAMEWORKS FOR THE EVALUATION OF OUTCOMES

The International Classification of Functioning, Disability, and Health (ICF) Model

The World Health Organization's International Classification of Functioning, Disability and Health (Fig. 3.1) (WHO 2019) and its pediatric equivalent, the ICF for Children and Youth (Simeonsson et al. 2003; ICF Browser) provide a unified language to classify health and health-related domains within a comprehensive framework to measure health outcomes associated with any health condition, (Simeonsson et al. 2003) including childhood-onset disability like CP (Ostensjø, Carlberg, and Vøllestad 2003; Majnemer and Mazer 2004). The ICF reflects a paradigm shift from a purely medical model to an integrated model of human functioning and disability that evaluates the impact of a health condition at three different domains/levels of functioning: (1) body functions/structure, (2) activities, and (3) participation. In the ICF framework, body structures refer to the anatomical structures directly or indirectly affected by the health condition of interest (e.g. brain, muscle, bone). Body functions refer to physiological functions of body systems (e.g. voluntary movement of a limb segment, strength, balance). Body functions and structures are typically necessary for activities which are specific tasks or actions (e.g. sitting, walking, running). The performance of these actions facilitate participation, which is doing the things that one wants to do to engage in life roles (e.g. going to school, playing sports), which in turn contributes to one's quality of life.

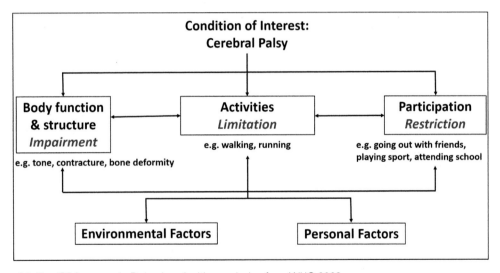

Figure 3.1 The ICF framework. Reproduced with permission from WHO 2002.

The impact of a health condition on the body structures (e.g. periventricular leukomalacia, muscle contracture, or excessive anteversion) and body functions (e.g. decreased range of motion or lever arm dysfunction) are the biophysical impairments that might lead to activity limitations, (e.g. inability to run), which might result in participation restrictions (e.g. inability to keep up with friends or play sports). The ICF framework also incorporates the influence of environmental factors, (e.g. home/school/community, socio-economic status, access to health care) and personal factors (e.g. culture, lifestyle preferences, motivation, and personality) (Majnemer 2012) which can exacerbate or mitigate limitations of activity and participation restrictions. These contextual factors explain the gap between one's capacity or what one can do and actual performance which is what one actually does do in daily life (Young et al. 1996).

Goldberg has previously proposed a framework of outcome assessments in which he made the distinction between the more immediate 'technical' outcomes of an intervention, (e.g. correction of equinus contracture following a gastrocnemius lengthening or correction of femoral anteversion following derotational osteotomy of the femur) from 'functional' outcomes which were the reasons for which the operation was being done (e.g. decreased tripping, improved endurance, correction of the internal rotation gait appearance) (1991). Our clinical interventions typically act at the level of body functions and structures or the biophysical impairments. For instance, botulinum neurotoxin A injections act at the level of the neuromuscular junction to block the release of acetylcholinesterase, while a selective dorsal rhizotomy involves something (cutting) some of the posterior nerve roots, both indirect means to achieve the technical outcome of reduced muscle tone. Multilevel orthopedic surgery addresses muscle contractures and bony deformities, the correction of which are the technical outcomes of our interventions. It is assumed that these technical outcomes will lead to the functional outcomes that patients and parents want, which might include improved activities and participation with fewer restrictions (Narayanan 2012). However, a technically successful outcome may not necessarily result in a functionally successful outcome. The latter are more meaningful to patients and parents, while the former are the means to that end. For Alex, a measurable reduction in the popliteal angle (after his medial hamstring lengthening) or normalization of the femoral anteversion (after the femoral derotational osteotomies) is of little relevance if his knees are still bent when he is walking and if he is still unable to keep up with his friends.

Nevertheless, it remains important to measure both technical outcomes at the level of the body functions/structures as well as the functional outcomes at the level of activities and participation, if only to understand how the former contributed to changes in the latter. It is important to recognize that a positive impact on activities and participation can be achieved without an intervention to correct impairments. For example, the use of powered mobility tools (wheelchair) might provide an alternative means of efficient locomotion, which may increase participation by allowing an individual to be independent and able to move around faster and with less effort. On the other hand, these gains in participation might be accompanied by a negative impact at the level of body function and structure, such as decreased cardiovascular fitness or increased knee flexion contractures.

The Priority Framework for Outcomes Evaluation

The Priority Framework is a useful way to conceptualize the relationship between patient problems, interventions, and outcomes of those interventions (Fig. 3.2) (Narayanan et al. 2005; Narayanan 2018). Alex has a lived experience with his cerebral palsy. Associated with this experience are the symptoms or problems he might encounter that might interfere with his life. His parents know him well and have their own sets of concerns about what the future might bring, based on their understanding of the natural history. Alex and his parents have a set of wishes and expectations that pertain to his condition. Patients' concerns about their health condition and or its treatments, their desires (wishes), and expectations of treatments collectively constitute patient priorities (Uhlmann, Inui, and Carter 1984; Kravitz et al. 1996; Narayanan 2018). The expression of these priorities or their elicitation by a clinician enables a patient to define a set of goals which can influence their choice or preference for specific treatments (Bowling and Ebrahim 2001).

There are multiple perspectives to consider. The priorities of the patient (child) may not be concordant with those of the parents. Clinicians have an important role to play in the conceptualization of these goals. Clinicians have knowledge about the natural history, as yet not experienced by the patient, and knowledge about the experiences of other patients that can inform patients' and parents' priorities and goals. Some patients or parents may not express their priorities and goals. It is, therefore, the responsibility of the clinician to seek outpatient and parent goals, even if they are not explicitly forthcoming. The clinician's evaluation of the patient includes objective assessments of the impairments at the level of the body functions/structure (e.g. gait analysis) that can contribute valuable insights. The elicitation of patients' priorities might unmask hitherto unexpressed patient preferences and expectations which in turn might influence shared decision making, allow for more informed consent about patient-specific treatments, and facilitate the evaluation of outcomes that matter most to patients (Entwistle et al. 1998).

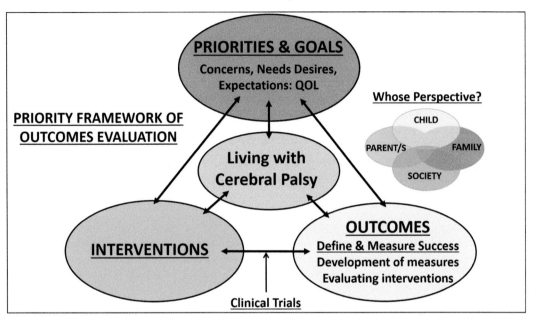

Figure 3.2 The Priority Framework for Outcomes Assessment. Reproduced with permission from Narayanan 2008.

Understanding priorities and goals are, therefore, crucial for making decisions about interventions that will best address these. What does Alex want? What do his parents want from surgery? If our interventions are intended to address these priorities and goals, their effectiveness must be evaluated using outcome measures that specifically incorporate the goals and priorities of the patient population (Narayanan 2018). Outcomes are most meaningful when they are aligned with patient priorities and goals. Did Alex and his parents get what they wanted or expected from his surgery? Were his goals met? Patient-based outcome measures will only be meaningful if the questions asked of patients reflect what's relevant and important to them (Amadio 1993; Wright, Rudicel, and Feinstein 1994). The Priority Framework ties together the concepts of patient priorities, choice of interventions to address those priorities, and evaluation of the success (or not) of those interventions based on outcomes that include patient priorities that can best judge whether those priorities were sufficiently addressed. Later in this chapter, we will discuss how we can use this framework in our evaluation of the appropriateness or relevance of different patient-reported outcome measures.

OUTCOME MEASURES: GENERAL CONSIDERATIONS

Patient-reported outcome measures (PROMs) are the criterion standard to evaluate the effectiveness of interventions. The content of PROMs should have been derived from patients themselves and in the case of children, parents, or caregivers as well. When the perspectives of patients are not accessible because they are very young or cognitively unable, one has to rely on the report of the child's parent/s. The views of older children can and must be taken into consideration, but their perspectives might differ from those of their parents. The level of agreement between parents and children is usually better for domains reflecting physical activity, functioning, and symptoms, but poorer for domains that reflect more social or emotional issues (Eiser and Morse 2001). Whenever possible, both perspectives should be considered during decision making and for measuring outcomes as well.

In addition to the perspective of patients and parents derived from PROMs, clinicians will also want to understand the technical outcomes of their intervention. The impact on targeted musculoskeletal impairments and objective gait-related outcomes (e.g. 3D gait analyses) are particularly important. These technical outcomes are crucial for understanding the reason for the success or failure of interventions, and their relationship to patient-reported outcomes. Clinicians should use these outcomes to continuously evaluate their treatment algorithms and intervention techniques. The knowledge derived from these assessments will allow clinicians to select the optimal type of treatment at each stage of motor development of the individual child and to fine-tune the selected treatment based on patient-specific data. These technical outcomes can facilitate longitudinal patient-tailored treatment planning. In the context of research, databases of such detailed outcome parameters may serve to better understand the relationship between technical outcomes and patient/parent experienced outcomes, to explore where these are closely linked, and to provide input for treatment prediction algorithms and objective intervention assessments.

Some outcomes might be more important than others, and different stakeholders will have different perspectives on the relative importance of different outcomes. In general, clinical outcomes are more relevant to patients and clinicians, while nonclinical outcomes including process measures (e.g. length of stay; cost-effectiveness) are of interest to hospital administrators, payers, and health policymakers.

OUTCOME MEASURES FOR AMBULATORY CEREBRAL PALSY

There are a number of assessment tools developed to measure outcomes in ambulatory CP. Each of these may cover one or more domains of the ICF framework. This section will provide an overview of the measures currently in use for ambulatory CP as well as research developments that are expected to bring new measures to the field. A first part will cover the technical measures of biophysical impairments that largely fall under the domain of body functions and structures. A second part will cover the patient-based and parent-reported outcomes that span the domains of activity and participation'

The appropriate measures to use depends on the purpose of the outcome measurement. Any measurement tool must have evidence of reliability (stable when no change has occurred) and validity (measure what is intended to be measured). Outcome measures are evaluative, and therefore should also be shown to be responsive or sensitive to change, when important change has occurred, either in a positive or negative direction (deterioration). In the following sections, an overview of outcome measures is provided. A combination of outcomes measures can be used for the PROMs as well as for previously described technical fine-tuning of patient-tailored treatment.

Technical Measures of Impairment

The heterogeneous and dynamic nature of CP is reflected in the variability of its clinical presentation, (Sussman et al. 2010) and the range of pathological movement patterns which evolve over time (Wren, Rethlefsen, and Kay 2005; Beckung et al. 2007; Riad, Haglund-Akerlind, and Miller 2007; Toro, Nester, and Farren 2007). This might explain the variability in reported treatment outcomes, with patients classifiable as good or bad responders (Schwartz 2013; Galarraga et al. 2017). The heterogeneity and change over time that characterizes CP requires longitudinal assessments of these impairments, which form the basis of our understanding of the underlying pathophysiology, and therefore the potential targets of our interventions. Treatment decisions should be patient-specific (Õunpuu 2015). These assessments allow us to better understand and plan the optimal timing and types of intervention/s for a specific patient, and also to measure the change (correction) of these impairments following the intervention. Therefore, these assessments are not only measures of the technical outcome but also serve as part of the continual monitoring of these dynamic impairments over the course of the child's development.

For each individual patient, the patient characteristics, such as age, topographic/severity classifications (GMFCS level), developmental history, comorbidities, treatment history must be ascertained along with current functional abilities and a list of physical symptoms and functional problems to provide context for the subsequent assessment that may facilitate the understanding of the source of these problems. Assessments include the physical examination of the musculoskeletal impairments complemented with data from diagnostic imaging, (Davids et al. 2004) and dynamic assessments, that include video imaging of walking as well as 3D gait analysis. These assessments can influence clinical decision-making and are also used to assess interventions' effects on gait (Cook et al. 2003; Lofterød and Terjesen 2008; Wren et al. 2013).

Physical Examination Measures

The standardized physical examination includes goniometric assessments of muscle length (range of motion), muscle tone quality (spasticity, dystonia) and intensity, muscle strength, bone alignment, and the degree of selective muscle control. These static assessments are at best complementary to and not always adequate proxies for the dynamic features of the child's gait, which can be assessed visually and by video or more objectively by gait analysis in a motion laboratory. For example, the Modified Ashworth Scale or the Tardieu scale can identify the presence of velocity-dependent hypertonia or spasticity, and quantify its severity to determine whether the patient might benefit from either local or systemic intervention/s to reduce muscle tone (e.g. to correct equinus gait). These scales can also be used to measure the reduction in tone following an intervention to determine whether the intervention was technically successful. Similarly, the immediate objectives of multilevel orthopedic surgery followed by a rehabilitation program are to optimize biomechanics by addressing the impairments, such as contractures of the gastrocnemius or the medial hamstrings; the lever arm dysfunction arising from the increased femoral anteversion; or the weakness of the quadriceps and hip extensor muscles. Following multilevel surgery, changes in range of motion, femoral anteversion, and muscle strength could be measured. However, improvements in these measures are merely indicators that the technical objectives of the operation were achieved, but are not in and of themselves, the outcomes that really matter to patients.

Visual/Video Gait Analysis

The collective impact of these static impairments on gait can be quantified using visual analysis with video and 3D gait analysis in a motion laboratory. The use of video, which requires minimal resources and is widely available, facilitates a more detailed visual examination of gait while capturing and recording this information for additional and repeated evaluation, and for comparison after an intervention (Borel,

Schneider, and Newman 2011). The ability to visualize gait in at least two separate planes (sagittal and frontal), even simultaneously if a split-screen option is available, and in slow-motion or frame by frame, allows for a more systematic multilevel and multi-planar evaluation. Various aspects or events of the gait cycle can be qualified and the deviations from normal quantified visually. The Edinburgh Visual Gait Score is generated by the use of a chart that documents seventeen distinct events (12 in stance phase; 5 in swing phase) involving the position of the foot, knee, hip, pelvis, and trunk in the sagittal, coronal, and transverse planes where applicable (Read et al. 2003). Each event is scored as normal (0), moderately (1), or markedly (2) deviated from normal, regardless of the direction of the deviation. The total score quantifies the overall deviation from normal, where normal would score '0'.

3D GAIT ANALYSIS

3D gait analysis has been generally accepted as the criterion standard to evaluate the dynamic nature of CP both to support clinical decision making and to evaluate treatment outcomes of gait objectively (Cook et al. 2003; Lofterød and Terjesen 2008; Wren et al. 2013). 3D gait analysis objectively quantifies the pathological motion patterns of the child with CP, allowing comparisons to typically developing children. Gait analysis generates kinematic and kinetic data, dynamic electromyography (EMG), and oxygen consumption, as well as useful spatiotemporal measures of walking speed, stride length, and cadence. The resulting data structure is highly dimensional and complex, often with quasi-periodic temporal dependence (cf. gait analysis waveforms) and time-dependency (e.g. gait patterns) (Chau 2001). This results in a comprehensive, patient-specific, multifaceted data set. These are used for pattern recognition and classification, clinical decision making, and also for evaluating the outcomes of interventions. Clinicians face many challenges associated with the extraction and analysis of information from the large amount of data.

The challenge of data reduction of the multifaceted data sets

A frequently applied data reduction approach in daily clinical practice is the study of clinically relevant gait features that are extracted from the continuous gait waveforms. These parameters represent discrete kinematic or kinetic variables, such as maximal joint angles reached throughout the full or part of the gait cycle, (Goldberg, Õunpuu, and Delp 2003; Wren, Rethlefsen, and Kay 2005; Wolf et al. 2006; Sangeux, Rodda, and Graham 2015; Nieuwenhuys et al. 2016; Gómez-Pérez et al. 2019) as well as spatiotemporal parameters. Unfortunately, although discrete parameterization of gait waveforms is frequently applied in clinical practice, it has some disadvantages. First, potentially important information might be lost as only a limited number of variables are extracted from the waveforms. Moreover, there is often a lack of agreement on the set of gait features that define a certain gait pattern, such as stiff knee (Goldberg, Õunpuu, and Delp 2003; Wren, Rethlefsen, and Kay 2005) or crouch gait (Rodda et al. 2004; Wren, Rethlefsen, and Kay 2005). Finally, the temporal nature of gait is overlooked in the discrete features, and the pattern of the gait curve is not taken into account (Chau 2001). The use of continuous gait features is an alternative approach to discrete features. These parameters usually focus on one (or more) clinically relevant section(s) of the gait cycle and describe the kinematics/kinetics of that phase (Zwick et al. 2004; Shorter et al. 2008).

The definition of gait features can be expert-driven when they are based on available clinical expert knowledge or on literature search; or can be data-driven, when they are defined using automatic data reduction techniques. The strength of expert-driven features is that they are more easily understood and accepted by clinicians. However, a pure expert-driven approach creates a set of features that are characterized by incompleteness and high risk for collinearity. When using such an incomplete set of features, interesting potential data, not (yet) detected by clinicians, may be lost. Moreover, a high reliance on features with unknown high collinearity may potentially result in the allocation of increased weight to certain problems, impeding clinical reasoning. The data-driven approach has applied several mathematical data reduction techniques to organize the rich high-dimensional 3D gait data sets into manageable formats. These include, amongst others, principal component analysis, cluster analysis, neural networks, wavelet transformation, self-organizing maps, and support vector machines (Lauer et al. 2005; Barton et al. 2006; Kirkwood et al. 2012; Mantovani et al. 2012; Meyer et al. 2015; Barton et al. 2019). The advantage of these methods is that they provide an objective, systematic, and structured approach to analyze gait data, and they result in complete and uncorrelated sets of features. Unfortunately, such approaches may also generate clinically irrelevant features and are therefore often not embraced by the clinical community (Nieuwenhuys et al. 2016).

Individual gait features have also been integrated into joint gait patterns, which represent combinations of discrete or continuous gait features of one or two joints. Such joint gait patterns follow specific categorization rules and have most frequently been defined for the ankle and knee joint (Schmidt-Rohlfing 2006; Benedetti et al. 2011; Van Gestel et al. 2011; Krzak et al. 2015; Sangeux, Rodda, and Graham 2015; Simon et al. 2015). However, recently, a comprehensive gait pattern system involving all lower limb joints, along with clear definitions of the motion patterns and the 3D gait analysis features characterizing these joint motion patterns, has been developed (Nieuwenhuys et al. 2016) and was found to be reliable (Nieuwenhuys et al. 2017) and valid (Nieuwenhuys et al. 2017a; Nieuwenhuys et al. 2017b). This gait pattern system was developed through a Delphi consensus study, where an international expert panel defined 49 joint patterns during gait, involving patterns for the pelvis, hip, knee, ankle, and foot in the sagittal, coronal, and transverse planes. Since these joint gait patterns were based on international experts' consensus (through the Delphi approach) (Nieuwenhuys et al. 2016), they are expected to be more easily understood by and acceptable to clinicians. Finally, data reduction has also been applied for musculoskeletal impairments, for example by creating composite scores on spasticity, or strength scores (Meyns et al. 2016; Chang et al. 2017).

Gait Analysis Derived Gait Indices

There are a number of multivariate statistical summary indices derived from instrumented 3D gait analysis that quantifies the overall magnitude of gait deviation from normal patterns. These measures not only serve to quantify the overall severity of gait differences but can be used to monitor progress and evaluate the effect of an intervention. The first of these was the Gillette Gait (Normalcy) Index (GGI), that quantifies the difference between a selected set of 16 discrete components of temporal-spatial and kinematic data of an individual from that of a normative data set, resulting in a single dimensionless measure that serves as a proxy for the overall gait pattern and has been shown to be reliable, discriminative, and sensitive to change following orthopedic interventions for CP (Schutte et al. 2000; Schwartz and Rozumalski 2008).

The Gait Deviation Index (GDI) is conceptually similar but addresses some of the limitations of the GGI, such as the arbitrary selection of the 16 discrete univariate parameters used and the non-normality of the index. The GDI is derived from the kinematic data (in 2% increments, or 51 points) of the gait cycle for nine kinematic variables (459 data points for each subject side), to produce a set of mutually independent joint rotation patterns of gait features that efficiently describe the overall gait pattern for each side. A reduced number of just 15 of these 459 gait features was shown to preserve 98% accurate reconstruction of the full data, and therefore sufficient to report the GDI that is scaled for easier interpretability (Schwartz and Rozumalski 2008). Every 10 points below 100 corresponds to one standard deviation away from the mean GDI for normal gait, and GDI ≥100 indicates the absence of gait pathology. The GDI is reportedly a superior multivariate measure of overall gait deviation and has demonstrated excellent face and concurrent validity (Schwartz and Rozumalski 2008).

The Gait Profile Score (GPS) is yet another single index measure that summarizes the overall deviation of kinematic gait data relative to normative data (Baker et al. 2009). Whereas the GDI is based on the difference (root mean square [RMS] distance) for just 15 gait features, the GPS is based on the root mean square difference taken over the same nine kinematic variables used in the GDI, but for the entire gait cycle. There is no additional scaling so that the final value is in degrees. The Gait Variable Scores is the RMS difference from average normal for each of the nine key component kinematic gait variables, which when combined for each side are presented as a Movement Analysis Profile (Beynon et al. 2010). This is useful because it provides additional information of the relative contribution of each of the kinematic variables to the overall deviation. The average of the RMS difference of all the Gait Variable Scores for a particular side will be equal to the GPS calculated from the entire gait vector. The GPS has high face validity (Beynon et al. 2010) and has also demonstrated concurrent validity with the Functional Abilities Questionnaire (FAQ), the GMFCS, GDI and GGI, (Baker et al. 2009) as well as with the GOAL questionnaire (Thomason et al. 2018).

Although these are valid measures of impairment at the ICF level of body function and structure, there are many limitations of relying on these indices as the primary outcome measure of effectiveness. These may contribute to but not necessarily correlate with the functional goals at the level of activities and participation that patients want (Abel et al. 2003). The kinematic data used are limited to nine variables, with some omitted because of inherent issues of quality and reliability around those variables. The trunk and upper extremities are not considered. Each of the kinematic variables used are weighted equally, when, in fact, the deviations of similar magnitude might have widely different levels of clinical importance. Similarly, the direction of the deviation is ignored (e.g. calcaneus is the same as equinus). Deviations recorded do not take into account whether these are primary or compensatory patterns, which are treated the same. These indices may, therefore, be good summary measures of the overall appearance of gait. However, even in this respect, it is important to acknowledge that these measures only apply to walking on level ground for a few meters in a motion lab, which may not be representative of overall gait function in the real world. Until such real-world gait analysis measures become available, there is an imperative for functional outcome measures that span the domains of activities and participation that matter more directly to patients and parents than degrees of movement of different limb segments.

Towards data integration

Nevertheless, since our treatments are most commonly performed at the impairment level, it is important to measure the effectiveness of those treatments at that level. These patients have a multifaceted disorder and different studies highlight the complex relationship between impairment and gait (Fosang and Baker 2006; Ross and Engsberg 2007; Eek and Beckung 2008; Dallmeijer et al. 2011; Eek, Tranberg, and Beckung 2011; Kim and Park 2011; Nieuwenhuys et al. 2017; Papageorgiou et al. 2019). To fine-tune patient-tailored interventions, the clinical team must be able to link the pathologic gait features to the levels of spasticity, muscle weakness, lack of muscle control, and/or secondary deformities (Baker et al. 2016). In order to satisfy our assumption that addressing these impairments will improve gait, (Dodd, Taylor, and Damiano 2002; Ross and Engsberg 2007; Sussman et al. 2010; Kim and Park 2011) the exploration of the link between the underlying impairments and gait features and patterns must continue, along with the link between gait features, in turn to patients' functional activities and participation. Improved insight into the interaction between neuromuscular impairments and gait and their impact on functional activities and participation may significantly influence the clinical decision-making process.

Functional and Patient Reported Outcome Measures
Gross Motor Function Measure (GMFM-66)

The GMFM is a widely used, validated observational measure of gross motor function in children with CP (Russell et al. 1989; Russell et al. 2000; Avery et al. 2003). The items of the GMFM span the child's gross motor functional skills across five dimensions: (1) lying and rolling; (2) sitting;

(3) crawling/kneeling; (4) standing; and (5) walking/running and jumping. A trained physiotherapist observes the independent achievement of these motor function tasks and assigns each task a score on a 4-point ordinal scale (0=does not initiate; 1=initiates <10% of activity; 2=partially completes 10% to <100% of activity; and 3=completes activity). Scores for each dimension (0 to 100) are a percentage of the maximum score for that dimension, and the total score (1 to 100) is obtained by the average of the scores of the five dimensions. The original GMFM, which had 88 items, has undergone Rasch analysis to develop the more efficient unidimensional and hierarchical scale, the GMFM-66, which improves the interpretability and clinical utility of the GMFM (Russell et al. 1989; Avery et al. 2003). These improvements include the ordering of the items according to difficulty, the interval properties of the scale, the decreased administration time, and a computer scoring system that calculates the total score and standard error even when some items are missing (Russell et al. 1989.) The GMFM has been used extensively in numerous intervention trials for ambulatory CP and has been shown to be sensitive to change following orthopedic surgery in ambulatory children with CP (Damiano, Gilgannon, and Abel 2005). Moreover, there are published data on population-based longitudinal changes in GMFM-66 scores over time for all five GMFCS levels of the children with cerebral palsy (Rosenbaum et al. 2002). These motor development curves provide an excellent basis to make judgments of clinically significant improvements in GMFM following interventions that must exceed what one would expect from the natural history (Fig. 3.3).

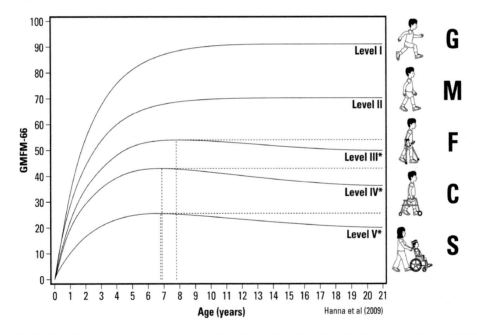

Figure 3.3 Predicted Average Development by the Gross Motor Function Classification System Levels (GMFCS). Adapted from Hanna et al. 2009.

The GMFM has many limitations. It is typically administered by a therapist who has to be trained to use the GMFM. It takes about one hour to complete and is typically performed in a clinical rather than real-world setting. Consequently, the GMFM is a measure of capacity or capability (observed under ideal circumstances) rather than actual performance, nor does it reveal how children might apply their motor function in the context of activities and participation in their daily life. It also does not take into account the quality of the functional activities.

Pediatric Outcomes Data Collection Instrument (PODCI)

The PODCI is a generic measure of musculoskeletal functional health outcomes reported by parents of children aged under 10 years, and by both parents and adolescents from 11 to 18-years old. The PODCI is comprised of 115 items spanning the domains of upper extremity function, transfers and mobility, sports and physical function, and comfort/pain. The PODCI generates a subscale score for each of these domains, the mean domain scores of which generate a Global Function score. The PODCI also includes items for happiness and satisfaction with physical condition; and expectations of treatment (Daltroy et al. 1998). Although it is reliable and valid for use in children with CP, (McCarthy et al. 2002) it has been shown to have only a modest sensitivity to change following orthopedic surgery in these children (Damiano, Gilgannon, and Abel 2005). It has many items that are less pertinent to ambulatory CP, such as those pertaining to upper extremity function. Furthermore, it has both floor and ceiling effects in various domains for this population (Harvey et al. 2008).

Gillette Functional Assessment Questionnaire (FAQ)

The FAQ is a self or proxy-report of ambulatory function that includes a ten-level ordinal rating scale of independent walking functional performance (FAQ Walking Scale) and 22 items of higher-level functional locomotor activities assessed for their degree of difficulty on a 5-level Likert-like scale (FAQ 22-item skill set). The FAQ Walking Scale has been shown to be a reliable and valid measure of functional walking status for children with disabilities, including CP (Novacheck, Stout, and Tervo 2000). The FAQ 22-item skill set provides information about higher-level skills. It demonstrates unidimensional structure of hierarchical skills related to locomotor function with no floor or ceiling effects (Gorton et al. 2011; Schwartz et al. 2004; Stout et al. 2008). The FAQ has been used to evaluate the effectiveness of orthopedic surgery in ambulatory children with CP (Novacheck, Trost, and Schwartz 2002; Tervo et al. 2002). Typically, only the FAQ Walking Scale is scored. The scoring and responsiveness of the FAQ 22-item skill set are less clear. There is a postintervention version of the FAQ which asks respondents to report perceived change in various domains following an intervention. However, eliciting responses about perceived change directly tied to an intervention increases the chance of a positive response bias. Some of the items in the postintervention version of the FAQ are technically worded (e.g. effect on 'body image'). The more appropriate format would be to evaluate the one's rating of each of these items at different time points (pre and post) without reference to the intervention.

Functional Mobility Scale (FMS)

The FMS measures the functional level of walking at 5m, 50m, and 500m, which correspond to walking distances associated with getting around in the home, school, and the wider community, respectively (Graham et al. 2004). For each of these three distances, the functional level is rated on an ordinal rating scale based on the level of walking aid that is required from the highest score of 6 (no walking aid required and no functional difficulty) to 1 (uses a wheelchair). The highest possible score is 6, 6, 6, and the lowest would be 1, 1, 1 for 5m, 50m, and 500m respectively. The FMS provides more granular information about the child's mobility than the GMFCS level. The FMS by self-report or proxy indicates the actual performance rather than capability, assessing what a child 'does do' in everyday life rather than what a child 'can do' in an idealized situation. The FMS captures only the level of walking aid required for different distances. It does not measure any of the other gait-related domains that are important to patients and their parents, such as the quality or appearance of the gait, or symptoms or problems associated with it, nor how these contribute to or hinder participation with activities that the child wants to do.

Patient-Reported Outcome Measurement Information System (PROMIS)

The National Institutes of Health, MD United States, has established PROMIS, an initiative to provide reliable, valid, flexible, precise, and responsive measures of patient-reported outcomes of physical, mental, and social health that can be accessed with through the assessment center (Gershon et al. 2010; PROMIS 2010). Large item banks are created for each domain of health (e.g. physical function; fatigue; pain; sleep/wake function; emotional distress; and social health), which evaluate the full spectrum of those domains (Cella et al. 2010). A number of child or proxy item banks are available for pediatric health domains (DeWitt et al. 2011; Irwin et al. 2012; Varni et al. 2012). Items are ordered and calibrated using item response theory, (Hambleton, Swaminathan, and Rogers 1991), which allows Computer Adaptive Testing (CAT) that can efficiently and precisely generate a domain score from a smaller subset of items administered by the computer-based on the respondent's earlier responses (Streiner, Norman, and Cairney 2015). Some of the PROMIS measures pertinent to ambulatory CP include the PROMIS Pediatric Mobility item bank, which assesses activities of physical mobility. The PROMIS Pain Intensity item pool assesses how much pain the person has experienced. The PROMIS Pain Interference item bank assesses the impact of pain on social, cognitive, emotional, physical, and recreational activities as well as sleep and enjoyment in life. The Peer Relationships item bank assesses the quality of relationships with friends and other acquaintances.

Pediatric Evaluation of Disability Inventory Computer Adaptive Test (PEDI-CAT)

The PEDI-CAT is an update of the PEDI instrument for children from birth to 21 years of age. The PEDI-CAT is a computer adaptive test that requires no special equipment other than software installed on a computer or tablet. It requires no physical testing. The PEDI-CAT evaluates ability in the same three functional areas as the PEDI (daily activities, mobility, and social/cognitive), but also has a fourth responsibility domain that reports the child's participation and amount of responsibility assumed for activities of daily living. The PEDI-CAT correlates well with previously validated instruments in patients with CP and is able to differentiate across both fine and gross motor functional levels (Dumas and Fragala-Pinkham 2012; Dumas et al. 2015; Dumas et al. 2017; Shore et al. 2017). The PEDI-CAT is a useful outcome instrument that can be used for any school-age child with a wide spectrum of disability.

Cerebral Palsy Computerized Adaptive Test (CP-CAT)

The CP-CAT has multiple scales of parent-reported outcomes that measure lower extremity function and mobility (LE CP-CAT), upper extremity function, activity and global health of children with CP, respectively (Haley et al. 2009; Haley et al. 2010; Gorton et al. 2010; Montpetit et al. 2011). The LE CP-CAT is based on a large bank of items that captures the level of lower extremity function based on the degree of difficulty (on a 5 point difficulty scale) associated with items that capture mobility, body transfers, ambulation with and without walking aids, and wheeled mobility (when applicable). The LE CP-CAT is scored on a T metric where the mean equals 50 and the standard deviation equals 10. The LE CP-CAT has good known-groups construct validity for ambulatory CP (scores decrease with increasing GMFCS level). The LE CP-CAT has been tested longitudinally for its responsiveness following orthopedic surgery and has been shown to be more sensitive to change than the PODCI (Mulcahey et al. 2015).

Although CATs such as those in PROMIS and the PEDI-CAT can increase the efficiency and reduce respondent burden, they do have some limitations. Since CATs can only work for unidimensional and hierarchical constructs, multidimensional constructs would require a CAT for each domain. Outcomes like health-related quality of life, where individual preferences play an important role, do not lend themselves to CATs. Furthermore, even condition-specific CATs like the LE-CPCAT are less sensitive to change in children who are at GMFCS level II (Mulcahey et al. 2015). It has been speculated that this might be because their item banks might not include some items that are relevant to functional mobility outcomes.

GAIT OUTCOMES ASSESSMENT LIST (GOAL) QUESTIONNAIRE

There are numerous limitations associated with the PROMs, as previously discussed. Some are generic measures and insufficiently sensitive for the population of children and youth with ambulatory CP. Others are specific to CP, but too narrow in their focus, neglecting many domains that are related to and impacted by gait. It is also plausible that patients and parents perceive overall improved outcomes that might arise from other domains, such as the appearance of gait and body image, that are not captured by those measures that focus on lower extremity physical function alone. None of these measures developed their content by asking children and adolescents with CP or their parents what was important to them. The GOAL questionnaire (Narayanan 2018) was developed specifically to address these limitations. The items of the GOAL were derived from iterative qualitative interviews of patients with ambulatory CP and their parents, using the Priority Framework (Fig. 3.2) to capture their gait-related priorities and goals. The 49 items of the GOAL questionnaire spans seven domains: (1) independence and activities of daily living; (2) gait function; (3) comfort and endurance; sports and recreation; (4) gait appearance; (5) use of mobility aids and braces; and (6) body image and self esteem. The GOAL generates a standardized total score and 7 domain scores, each from 0 to 100. There is a child and parent version of the GOAL. For each item, the respondent not only indicates their level of performance but also whether making an improvement on that item is an important goal for them. This unique feature allows patient's and parents' treatment goals to be identified. These can identify patient expectations, including those that may not be realistic, and better inform shared decision making about the choice of interventions while serving as a more meaningful goal-based measure of outcomes for gait-related interventions. The GOAL is reliable and internally consistent. It has been shown to have construct and concurrent validity with strong correlations with the GPS, FMS, and FAQ (Thomason et al. 2018). If shown to be sensitive to change or responsive following an intervention, it has the potential to be a more meaningful and comprehensive functional outcome measure that spans the patient-centered domains of the ICF, including activities, participation, environmental and personal contextual factors aligned with the priorities and goals of this population. The GOAL questionnaire applied to Alex would suggest that from his perspective or that of his parents, the multilevel surgery has made him better in some domains, but not (perhaps yet) as much in others. He achieved his goals to walk with his feet flat on the ground and pointing straight ahead, to stop his knees rubbing against each other, and he is no longer tripping. However, he is still relying on his walker for support and has to wear the AFOs that he was hoping to avoid. The benefits have also come at the price of new symptoms of discomfort in his feet that are bothersome. The GOAL questionnaire is currently the only PROM that would capture all these elements.

OUTCOMES AS INPUT FOR TREATMENT PREDICTION ALGORITHMS

Treatments in ambulatory CP have been associated with variable outcomes, perhaps due to the heterogeneity of the population. There is a need for a better understanding of the source of patients' variable response to treatment, which would be crucial for the development of patient-specific prediction algorithms that can support clinicians in their decision-making process. Statistical models and machine learning techniques, such as regression models, Random Forest Algorithms, Support Vector Machines and Linear Discriminant Analysis, have been developed based on large patient cohorts and applied to predict treatment outcomes (Schwartz et al. 2013; Ries, Novacheck, and Schwartz 2014; Schwartz, Rozumalski, and Novacheck 2014; Funk et al. 2015; Oudenhoven et al. 2019). These models most commonly use a selection of the patient-specific data to predict the probability that a specific treatment would be successful. The most frequently used outcome parameters as input for prediction algorithms are derived from gait analysis, sometimes combined with physical examination of musculoskeletal impairments (Schwartz, Rozumalski, and Novacheck 2014; Funk et al. 2015) and patient characteristics (Funk et al. 2015; Oudenhoven et al. 2019). The majority of the statistical models predict the success of treatment as a binary outcome ('good' or 'bad' responders), based on one (often an overall gait deviation index) or a few gait parameters (e.g. specific joint angles). Such an approach may not adequately represent the real-world outcomes and almost certainly fail to capture a more holistic view of the patient status. There is an imperative to study both the technical and patient-reported outcomes and to explore the relationship between these for specific patients, so that prediction algorithms may become more clinically relevant when the observed changes are placed in the context of patient-specific expected changes.

CHALLENGES OF MEASURING OUTCOMES IN AMBULATORY CP

There are many challenges to evaluating meaningful outcomes in children with chronic conditions such as ambulatory CP.

1. Although there are many patient (or parent) reported outcome measures, their content may not adequately represent patients' or parents' priorities and goals.
2. When working with children, whose goals should prevail? It is important to measure the goals of children and their parents whenever possible. For a chronic condition, the perspective of the child when cognitively able is important because he or she knows best about their own lived experience. The parents' perspectives are also important as they are the primary decision-makers and also more likely to have a long-term view. When children are young or cognitively impaired, we must rely on the priorities of their parents or the primary caregivers who know the child best.
3. Few PROMs have been tested for their responsiveness or sensitivity to change. Consequently, it is a challenge to interpret whether the lack of a difference following intervention is indicative of the ineffectiveness of the treatment or the unresponsiveness of the outcome measure, or both.
4. In ambulatory CP, the goals of our interventions might not always be reactive. Some interventions might be prophylactic in that they are intended to prevent some problem in the future. A prophylactic intervention will not be associated with a change or improvement in a PROM. For instance, gait-related interventions for adolescents with ambulatory CP might not appear to be effective because they are not associated with significant functional changes from baseline. The gross motor function curves begin to decline somewhat during adolescence (Fig. 3.4) (Hanna et al. 2009). Under those circumstances, preserving ambulatory function should be considered a successful outcome relative to the expected deterioration associated with the untreated natural history. Of course, this can only be ascertained if studies for this population include a comparison group to contrast treatment outcomes against natural history (Fig. 3.4).
5. On the other hand, at the younger end of the spectrum, all children with CP are expected to make functional gains up to the age of 6 or 7 years. Any intervention applied during this younger age range might appear to be effective. However, evidence of effectiveness should only be inferred if the improvement in functional outcome is greater than that expected from the natural history (Fig. 3.4). This speaks once again to the importance of a control group of untreated patients.

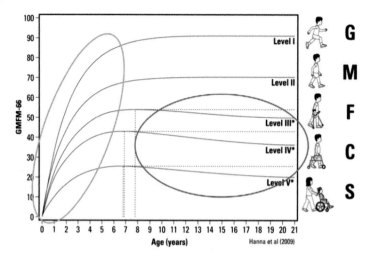

Figure 3.4 Natural history and the implication of timing of interventions on functional outcomes. Adapted from Hanna et al. 2009.

6. In certain situations, some patients might be asymptomatic, while others might be symptomatic at baseline (e.g. progressive hip displacement in CP). In a study evaluating the effectiveness of an intervention for such a condition, the inclusion of both symptomatic and asymptomatic patients in the analysis might lead to an underestimation of benefit. The apparent lack of response in the asymptomatic group might dilute any improvements noted in the symptomatic group. This could lead to an underestimation of the true effect unless the asymptomatic and symptomatic groups are identified and stratified at baseline so that they can be analyzed separately.

7. Rigorous assessment of clinical outcomes is essential to evaluate the effectiveness of treatments. It is challenging to handle the comprehensive longitudinal data set of ambulatory patients with CP, including gait analysis data, musculoskeletal impairment data, patient characteristics, and then to dose intervention by clinical expert knowledge. Data reduction is needed but should be balanced: enough (i.e. not too detailed, such that it remains manageable), and not too much (i.e. detailed enough to provide a complete picture).

8. The value of clinical judgment and experience that arises from qualitative evaluations of complex multifaceted data by clinicians must not be underestimated. However, these judgments are difficult to quantify or generalize and not necessarily consistent or dependably correct. Purely objective approaches like machine learning have not yet been clinically embraced. Clinical expertise and judgment needs to be embedded into data-driven decision-making algorithms.

CONCLUSION

There are a myriad of complementary or competing treatment strategies for ambulatory CP, with wide variations in practice with respect to the timing, dosing, and combination of treatments that are recommended. Much work remains to be done to evaluate the effectiveness (or not) of these interventions and treatment strategies. The sheer number, diversity, complexity, and costs of treatment options provide a compelling imperative for comparative effectiveness research to generate much-needed evidence to justify any of these treatments. Clinical trials and prospective comparative cohort studies will be of little value without the appropriate outcome measures to define more meaningfully what 'works' for patients (Entwistle et al. 1998). This chapter provides a framework to understand the scope of outcomes that we must consider and an overview of the current and emerging outcome measures that we can use to make judgments about interventions for ambulatory CP.

PRIORITIES FOR NEXT 5-YEARS & BEYOND

- Define variables of interest that are critically associated with functional gait and related to patient priorities and goals.
- Identify optimal set of responsive and goal-oriented technical, observed, and patient/parent reported outcome measures that will comprehensively evaluate the effectiveness of gait related interventions.
- Develop portable and other technologies to expand data capture of gait and more broadly functional activities in the real world.
- Expand the utilization of computer adaptive testing platforms to enhance our ability to capture outcomes on our patients more efficiently.
- Promote the use of goal-based PROMs that might facilitate shared decision making as well as outcome assessment.
- Establish multicentre databases that collect standardized sets of core outcomes that include prognostic and predictive variables and meaningful outcome measures, which will facilitate data pooling across multiple centers to support the development of improved prognostic or prediction algorithms and patient-tailored decision making.
- Facilitate individualized patient-specific treatment decision making using machine learning approaches and other novel, efficient and computationally feasible statistical algorithms for the analysis of multi-dimensional data characterizing ambulatory CP combined with the extraction and implementation of clinical expert knowledge.

REFERENCES

Abel MF, Damiano DL, Blanco JS, et al. (2003) Relationships among musculoskeletal impairments and functional health status in ambulatory cerebral palsy. *J Pediatr Orthop* **23**: 535–541.

Amadio PC (1993) Outcomes measurements. *J Bone Joint Surg Am* **75**: 1583–1584.

Avery LM, Russell DJ, Raina PS, Walter SD, Rosenbaum PL (2003) Rasch analysis of the gross motor function measure: validating the assumptions of the rasch model to create an interval-level Measure. *Arch Phys Med Rehabil* **84**: 697–705.

Baker R, Esquenazi A, Benedetti MG, Desloovere K (2016) Gait analysis: Clinical facts. *Eur J Phys Rehabil Med* **52**: 560–574.

Baker R, McGinley JL, Schwartz MH, et al. (2009) The gait profile score and movement analysis. *Gait Posture* **30**: 265–269.

Barton G, Lees A, Lisboa P, Attfield S (2006) Visualisation of gait data with Kohonen self-organising neural maps. *Gait Posture* **24**: 46–53.

Barton GJ, Hawken MB, Scott MA, Schwartz MH (2019) Leaving hip rotation out of a conventional 3D gait model improves discrimination of pathological gait in cerebral palsy: A novel neural network analysis. *Gait Posture* **70**: 48–52.

Beckung E, Carlsson G, Carlsdotter S, Uvebrant P (2007) The natural history of gross motor development in children with cerebral palsy aged 1 to 15 years. *Dev Med Child Neurol* **49**: 751–756.

Benedetti MG, D'Apote G, Faccioli S, Costi S, Ferrari A (2011) Equinus foot classification in cerebral palsy: An agreement study between clinical and gait analysis assessment. *Eur J Phys Rehabil Med* **47**: 213–221.

Beynon S, McGinley JL, Dobson F, Baker R. (2010) Correlations of the Gait Profile Score and the Movement Analysis Profile relative to clinical judgments. *Gait Posture* **32**: 129–132.

Borel S, Schneider P, Newman CJ (2011) Video analysis software increases the interrater reliability of video gait assessments in children with cerebral palsy. *Gait and Posture* **33**: 727–729.

Bowling A, Ebrahim S (2001) Measuring patients' preferences for treatment and perceptions of risk. *Qual Health Care* **10 Suppl 1**: i2–8.

Cella D, Riley W, Stone A et al. (2010) The Patient-Reported Outcomes Measurement Information System (PROMIS) developed and tested its first wave of adult self-reported health outcome item banks: 2005-2008. *J Clin Epidemiol* **63**: 1179–1194.

Chang CH, Chen YY, Yeh KK, Chen CL (2017) Gross motor function change after multilevel soft tissue release in children with cerebral palsy. *Biomed J* **40**: 163–168.

Chau T (2001) A review of analytical techniques for gait data. Part 1: Fuzzy, statistical and fractal methods. *Gait Posture* **13**: 49–66.

Chau T (2001) A review of analytical techniques for gait data. Part 2: Neural network and wavelet methods. *Gait Posture* **13**: 102–120.

Cook RE, Schneider I, Hazlewood ME, Hillman SJ, Robb JE (2003) Gait analysis alters decision-making in cerebral palsy. *J Pediatr Orthop* **23**: 292–295.

Dallmeijer AJ, Baker R, Dodd KJ, Taylor NF (2011) Association between isometric muscle strength and gait joint kinetics in adolescents and young adults with cerebral palsy. *Gait Posture* **33**: 326–332.

Daltroy LH, Liang MH, Fossel AH, Goldberg MJ (1998) The POSNA pediatric musculoskeletal functional health questionnaire: report on reliability, validity, and sensitivity to change. Pediatric Outcomes Instrument Development Group. Pediatric Orthopaedic Society of North America. *J Pediatr Orthop.* **18**: 561–571.

Damiano DL, Gilgannon MD, Abel MF (2005) Responsiveness and uniqueness of the pediatric outcomes data collection instrument compared to the gross motor function measure for measuring orthopaedic and neurosurgical outcomes in cerebral palsy. *J Pediatr Orthop* **25**: 641–645.

Davids JR, Ounpuu S, DeLuca PA, Davis RB (2004) Optimization of walking ability of children with cerebral palsy. *Instr Course Lect* **53**: 511–522.

DeWitt EM, Stucky BD, Thissen D et al. (2011) Construction of the eight-item patient-reported outcomes measurement information system pediatric physical function scales: built using item response theory. *J Clin Epidemiol* **64**: 794–804.

Dodd KJ, Taylor NF, Damiano DL (2002) A systematic review of the effectiveness of strength-training programs for people with cerebral palsy. *Arch Phys Med Rehabil* **83**: 1157–1164.

Dumas HM, Fragala-Pinkham MA (2012) Concurrent Validity and Reliability of the Pediatric Evaluation of Disability Inventory-Computer Adaptive Test Mobility Domain. *Pediatr Phys Ther* **24**: 171–176.

Dumas HM, Fragala-Pinkham MA, Rosen EL, Lombard KA, Farrell C (2015) Pediatric Evaluation of Disability Inventory Computer Adaptive Test (PEDI-CAT) and Alberta Infant Motor Scale (AIMS): Validity and Responsiveness. *Phys Ther* **95**: 1559–1568.

Dumas HM, Fragala-Pinkham MA, Rosen EL, O'Brien JE (2017) Construct validity of the pediatric evaluation of disability inventory computer adaptive test (PEDI-CAT) in children with medical complexity. *Disabil Rehabil* **39**: 2446–2451.

Eek MN, Beckung E (2008) Walking ability is related to muscle strength in children with cerebral palsy. *Gait Posture* **28**: 366–371.

Eek MN, Tranberg R, Beckung E (2011) Muscle strength and kinetic gait pattern in children with bilateral spastic CP. *Gait Posture* **33**: 333–337.

Eiser C, Morse R (2001) Can parents rate their child's health-related quality of life? Results of a systematic review. *Qual Life Res.* **10**: 347–357.

Entwistle VA, Renfrew MJ, Yearley S, Forrester J, Lamont T (1998) Lay perspectives: advantages for health research. *BMJ* **316**: 463–466.

Fosang A, Baker R (2006) A method for comparing manual muscle strength measurements with joint moments during walking. *Gait Posture* **24**: 406–411.

Funk JF, Panthen A, Bakir MS et al. (2015) Predictors for the benefit of selective dorsal rhizotomy. *Res Dev Disabil* **37**: 127–134.

Galarraga COA, Vigneron V, Dorizzi B, Khouri N, Desailly E (2017) Predicting postoperative gait in cerebral palsy. *Gait Posture* **52**: 45–51.

Gershon RC, Rothrock N, Hanrahan R, Bass M, Cella D (2010) The use of PROMIS and assessment center to deliver patient-reported outcome measures in clinical research. *J Appl Meas* **11**: 304–314.

Goldberg MJ (1991) Measuring outcomes in cerebral palsy. *J Pediatr Orthop* **11**: 682–685.

Goldberg SR, Õunpuu S, Delp SL (2003) The importance of swing-phase initial conditions in stiff-knee gait. *J Biomech* **36**: 1111–1116.

Gómez-Pérez C, Font-Llagunes JM, Martori JC, Vidal Samsó J (2019) Gait parameters in children with bilateral spastic cerebral palsy: a systematic review of randomized controlled trials. *Dev Med Child Neurol* **61**: 770–782.

Gorton GE 3rd, Stout JL, Bagley AM, Bevans K, Novacheck TF, Tucker CA (2011) Gillette Functional Assessment Questionnaire 22-item skill set: factor and Rasch analyses. *Dev Med Child Neurol* **53**: 250–255.

Gorton GE 3rd, Watson K, Tucker CA, Tian F, Montpetit K, Haley SM, Mulcahey MJ (2010) Precision and content range of a parent-reported item bank assessing lower extremity and mobility skills in children with cerebral palsy. *Dev Med Child Neurol* **52**: 660–665.

Graham HK, Harvey A, Rodda J, Nattrass GR, Pirpiris M (2004) The Functional Mobility Scale (FMS). *J Pediatr Orthop* **24**: 514–520.

Haley SM, Chafetz RS, Tian F, Montpetit K, Watson K, Gorton G, Mulcahey MJ (2010) Validity and reliability of physical functioning computer-adaptive tests for children with cerebral palsy. *J Pediatr Orthop* **30**: 71–75.

Haley SM, Ni P, Dumas HM et al. (2009) Measuring global physical health in children with cerebral palsy: illustration of a multidimensional bi-factor model and computerized adaptive testing. *Qual Life Res* **18**: 359–370.

Hambleton RK, Swaminathan H, Rogers HJ (1991) *Fundamentals of Item Response Theory*. New York: Sage Publications.

Hanna SE, Rosenbaum PL, Bartlett DJ et al. (2009) Stability and decline in gross motor function among children and youth with cerebral palsy aged 2 to 21 years. *Dev Med Child Neurol* **51**: 295–302.

Harvey A, Robin J, Morris ME, Graham HK (2008) A systematic review of measures of activity limitation for children with cerebral palsy. *Devp Med Child Neurol* **50**: 190–198.

ICF Browser. http://apps.who.int/classifications/icfbrowser/Default.aspx. Accessed March 10, 2020.

Irwin DE, Gross HE, Stucky BD, et al. (2012) Development of six PROMIS pediatrics proxy-report item banks. *Health Qual Life Outcomes* **10**: 22.

Kim WH, Park EY (2011) Causal relation between spasticity, strength, gross motor function, and functional outcome in children with cerebral palsy: A path analysis. *Dev Med Child Neurol* **53**: 68–73.

Kirkwood RN, Franco RDLLD, Furtado SC, Barela AMF, Deluzio KJ, Mancini MC (2012) Frontal Plane Motion of the Pelvis and Hip during Gait Stance Discriminates Children with Diplegia Levels I and II of the GMFCS. *ISRN Pediatr* **2012**: 163039.

Kravitz RL, EJ Callahan, Paterniti D Antonius D, Dunham M, Lewis CE (1996) Prevalence and sources of patients' unmet expectations for care. *Ann Intern Med* **125**: 730–737.

Krzak JJ, Corcos DM, Damiano DL, et al. (2015) Kinematic foot types in youth with equinovarus secondary to hemiplegia. *Gait Posture* **41**: 402–408.

Lauer RT, Stackhouse C, Shewokis PA, Smith BT, Orlin M, McCarthy JJ (2005) Assessment of wavelet analysis of gait in children with typical development and cerebral palsy. *J Biomech* **38**: 1351–1357.

Lofterød B, Terjesen T (2008) Results of treatment when orthopaedic surgeons follow gait-analysis recommendations in children with CP. *Dev Med Child Neurol.* **50**: 503–509.

Majnemer A (2012) *Measures for Children with Developmental Disabilities an ICF-CY Approach*. London: Mac Keith Press.

Majnemer A, Mazer B (2004) New directions in the outcome evaluation of children with cerebral palsy. *Semin Pediatr Neurol* **11**: 11–17.

Mantovani G, Lamontagne M, Varin D, Cerulli GG, Beaulé PE (2012) Comparison of total hip arthroplasty surgical approaches by Principal Component Analysis. *J Biomech* **45**: 2109–2115.

McCarthy ML, Silberstein CE, Atkins EA, Harryman SE, Sponseller PD, Hadley-Miller NA (2002) Comparing reliability and validity of pediatric instruments for measuring health and well-being of children with spastic cerebral palsy. *Dev Med Child Neurol* **44**: 468–476.

Meyer CAG, Corten K, Fieuws S, et al. (2015) Biomechanical gait features associated with hip osteoarthritis: Towards a better definition of clinical hallmarks. *J Orthop Res* **33**: 1498–1507.

Meyns P, Van Gestel L, Leunissen I, et al. (2016) Macrostructural and Microstructural Brain Lesions Relate to Gait Pathology in Children with Cerebral Palsy. *Neurorehabil Neural Repair* 30: 817–833.

Montpetit K, Haley S, Bilodeau N, Ni P, Tian F, Gorton G 3rd, Mulcahey MJ (2011) Content range and precision of a computer adaptive test of upper extremity function for children with cerebral palsy. *Phys Occup Ther Pediatr* **31**: 90–102.

Mulcahey MJ, Slavin MD, Ni P et al. (2015) Computerized Adaptive Tests Detect Change Following Orthopaedic Surgery in Youth with Cerebral Palsy. *J Bone Joint Surg Am* **97**: 1482–1494.

Narayanan UG (2018) GOAL Questionnaire. https://lab.research.sickkids.ca/pscoreprogram/goal/

Narayanan UG (2012) Management of children with ambulatory cerebral palsy: an evidence based review. *J Pediatr Orthop* **32**: S172–181.

Narayanan UG (2018) Priority Based Scales for Children's Outcomes – Research & Evaluation (PSCORE) Program. https://lab.research.sickkids.ca/pscoreprogram/. Accessed March 10, 2020.

Narayanan UG, Wright JG, Hedden DM et al. (2005) Concerns, Desires and Expectations of Surgery for Adolescent Idiopathic Scoliosis: A Comparison of Patients', Parents' and Surgeons' Perspectives. *Orthopaedic Proceedings* **87-B**: 295–296.

Natsch S, Kullberg BJ, Hekster YA, van der Meer JWM (2003) Selecting outcome parameters in studies aimed at improving rational use of antibiotics - practical considerations. *J Clin Pharm Ther* **28**: 475–478.

Nieuwenhuys A, Õunpuu S, Van Campenhout A, et al. (2016) Identification of joint patterns during gait in children with cerebral palsy: A Delphi consensus study. *Dev Med Child Neurol* **58**: 306–313.

Nieuwenhuys A, Papageorgiou E, Desloovere K, Molenaers G, De Laet T (2017) Statistical parametric mapping to identify differences between consensus-based joint patterns during gait in children with cerebral palsy. *PLoS One* **12**: e0169834.

Nieuwenhuys A, Papageorgiou E, Molenaers G, Monari D, De Laet T, Desloovere K (2017) Inter- and intrarater clinician agreement on joint motion patterns during gait in children with cerebral palsy. *Dev Med Child Neurol* **59**: 750–755.

Nieuwenhuys A, Papageorgiou E, Pataky T, De Laet T, Molenaers G, Desloovere K (2016) Literature Review and Comparison of Two Statistical Methods to Evaluate the Effect of Botulinum Toxin Treatment on Gait in Children with Cerebral Palsy. *PLoS One* **11**: e0152697.

Nieuwenhuys A, Papageorgiou E, Schless S-H, De Laet T, Molenaers G, Desloovere K (2017) Prevalence of joint gait patterns defined by a Delphi consensus study is related to gross motor function, topographical classification, weakness, and spasticity, in children with cerebral palsy. *Front Hum Neurosci* **11**: 185.

Novacheck TF, Stout JL, Tervo R (2000) Reliability and validity of the Gillette Functional Assessment Questionnaire as an outcome measure in children with walking disabilities. *J Pediatr Orthop*. **20**: 75–81.

Novacheck TF, Trost JP, Schwartz MH (2002) Intramuscular psoas lengthening improves dynamic hip function in children with cerebral palsy. *J Pediatr Orthop* **22**: 158–164.

Ostensjø S, Carlberg EB, Vøllestad NK (2003) Everyday functioning in young children with cerebral palsy: functional skills, caregiver assistance, and modifications of the environment. *Dev Med Child Neurol* **45**: 603–612.

Oudenhoven LM, van der Krogt MM, Romei M et al. (2019) Factors Associated With Long-Term Improvement of Gait After Selective Dorsal Rhizotomy. *Arch Phys Med Rehabil* **100**: 474–480.

Õunpuu S, Gorton G, Bagley A, Sison-Williamson M, Hassani S, Johnson B, Oeffinger D (2015) Variation in kinematic and spatiotemporal gait parameters by Gross Motor Function Classification System level in children and adolescents with cerebral palsy. *Dev Med Child Neurol* **57**: 955–962.

Papageorgiou E, Simon-Martinez C, Guy Molenaers, Ortibus E, Van Campenhout A, Desloovere K (2019) Are spasticity, weakness, selectivity, and passive range of motion related to gait deviations in children with spastic cerebral palsy? A statistical parametric mapping study. *PLoS One* **14**: e0223363.

PROMIS: Patient Reported Outcomes Measurement Information System. http://www.healthmeasures.net/explore-measurement-systems/promis. Published 2010. Accessed March 10, 2020.

Read HS, Hazlewood ME, Hillman SJ, Prescott RJ, Robb JE (2003) Edinburgh Visual Gait Score for use in cerebral palsy. *Journal of Pediatric Orthopaedics* **23**: 296–301.

Riad J, Haglund-Akerlind Y, Miller F (2007) Classification of spastic hemiplegic cerebral palsy in children. *J Pediatr Orthop* **27**: 758–764.

Ries AJ, Novacheck TF, Schwartz MH (2014) A data driven model for optimal orthosis selection in children with cerebral palsy. *Gait Posture* **40**: 539–544.

Rodda JM, Graham HK, Carson L, Galea MP, Wolfe R. Sagittal gait patterns in spastic diplegia (2004) *J Bone Joint Surg Br* **86**: 251–258.

Rosenbaum PL, Walter SD, Hanna SE et al. (2002) Prognosis for gross motor function in cerebral palsy. Creation of motor development curves. *JAMA* **288**: 1357–1363.

Russell DJ, Avery LM, Rosenbaum PL, Raina PS, Walter SD, Palisano RJ (2000) Improved scaling of the gross motor function measure for children with cerebral palsy: evidence of reliability and validity. *Phys Ther* **80**: 873–885.

Russell DJ, Rosenbaum PL, Cadman DT, Gowland C, Hardy S, Jarvis S (1989) The gross motor function measure: a means to evaluate the effects of physical therapy. *Dev Med Child Neurol* **31**: 341–352.

Sangeux M, Rodda J, Graham HK (2015) Sagittal gait patterns in cerebral palsy: The plantarflexor-knee extension couple index. *Gait Posture* **41**: 586–591.

Schmidt-Rohlfing B, Bergamo F, Williams S, Rau G, Niethard F, Disselhorst-Klug C (2006) Interpretation of Surface EMGs in Children with Cerebral Palsy: An Initial Study Using a Fuzzy Expert System. *J Orthop Res Sept* **24**: 438–447.

Schutte LM, Narayanan U, Stout JL, Selber P, Gage JR, Schwartz MH (2000) An index for quantifying deviations from normal gait. *Gait Posture* **11**: 25–31.

Schwartz MH, Rozumalski A (2008) The gait deviation index: A new comprehensive index of gait pathology. *Gait Posture* **28**: 351–357.

Schwartz MH, Rozumalski A, Truong W, Novacheck TF (2013) Predicting the outcome of intramuscular psoas lengthening in children with cerebral palsy using preoperative gait data and the random forest algorithm. *Gait Posture* **37**: 473–479.

Schwartz MH, Rozumalski A, Novacheck TF (2014) Femoral derotational osteotomy: Surgical indications and outcomes in children with cerebral palsy. *Gait Posture* **39**: 778–783.

Schwartz MH, Viehweger E, Stout J, Novacheck TF, Gage JR (2004) Comprehensive treatment of ambulatory children with cerebral palsy: an outcome assessment. *J Pediatr Orthop* **24**: 45–53.

Shore BJ, Allar BG, Miller PE, Matheney TH, Snyder BD, Fragala-Pinkham MA (2017) Evaluating the Discriminant Validity of the Pediatric Evaluation of Disability Inventory: Computer Adaptive Test in Children With Cerebral Palsy. *Phys Ther* **97**: 669–676.

Shorter KA, Polk JD, Rosengren KS, Hsiao-Wecksler ET (2008) A new approach to detecting asymmetries in gait. *Clin Biomech* **23**: 459–467.

Simeonsson RJ, Leonardi M, Lollar D, Bjorck-Akesson E, Hollenweger J, Martinuzzi A (2003) Applying the International Classification of Functioning, Disability and Health (ICF) to measure childhood disability. *Disabil Rehabil* **25**: 602–610.

Simon AL, Ilharreborde B, Megrot F, et al. (2015) A descriptive study of lower limb torsional kinematic profiles in children with spastic diplegia. *J Pediatr Orthop* **35**: 576–582.

Stout JL, Gage JR, Schwartz MH, Novacheck TF (2008) Distal femoral extension osteotomy and patellar tendon advancement to treat persistent crouch gait in cerebral palsy. *J Bone Joint Surg Am* **90**: 2470–2484.

Streiner DL, Norman GR, Cairney J (2015) *Health Measurement Scales*. Vol 1. Oxford: Oxford University Press.

Sussman MD, Gage JR, Schwartz MH, Koop SE, Novacheck TF (2010) The Identification and Treatment of Gait Problems in Cerebral Palsy. *J Child Orthop* **4**: 177–178.

Tervo RC, Azuma S, Stout J, Novacheck T (2002) Correlation between physical functioning and gait measures in children with cerebral palsy. *Dev Med Child Neurol* **44**: 185–190.

Thomason P, Tan A, Donnan A, Rodda J, Graham HK, Narayanan U (2018) The Gait Outcomes Assessment List (GOAL): validation of a new assessment of gait function for children with cerebral palsy. *Dev Med Child Neurol* **60**: 618–623.

Toro B, Nester CJ, Farren PC (2007) Cluster analysis for the extraction of sagittal gait patterns in children with cerebral palsy. *Gait Posture* **25**: 157–165.

Trost JP, Schwartz MH, Krach LE, Dunn ME, Novacheck TF (2008) Comprehensive short-term outcome assessment of selective dorsal rhizotomy. *Dev Med Child Neurol* **50**: 765–71.

Uhlmann RF, Inui TS, Carter WB (1984) Patient requests and expectations. Definitions and clinical applications. *Med Care* **22**: 681–685.

Van Gestel L, De Laet T, Di Lello E, et al. (2011) Probabilistic gait classification in children with cerebral palsy: A Bayesian approach. *Res Dev Disabil* **32**: 2542–2552.

Varni JW, Thissen D, Stucky BD et al. (2012) PROMIS® Parent Proxy Report Scales: an item response theory analysis of the parent proxy report item banks. *Qual Life Res* **21**: 1223–1240.

WHO | International Classification of Functioning, Disability and Health (ICF) (2019) *WHO* https://www.who.int/classifications/icf/en/. Accessed March 10, 2020.

Wolf S, Loose T, Schablowski M, Do L, Ju H (2006) Automated feature assessment in instrumented gait analysis. *Gait Posture* **23**: 331–338.

Wren TAL, Elihu KJ, Mansour S, et al. (2013) Differences in implementation of gait analysis recommendations based on affiliation with a gait laboratory. *Gait Posture* **37**: 206–209.

Wren TAL, Rethlefsen S, Kay RM (2005) Prevalence of Specific Gait Abnormalities in Children With Cerebral Palsy Influence of Cerebral Palsy Subtype, Age, and Previous Surgery. *J Pediatr Orthop* **25**: 79–83.

Wright JG, Rudicel S, Feinstein AR (1994) Ask patients what they want. Evaluation of individual complaints before total hip replacement. *J Bone Joint Surg Br* **76**: 229–234.

Young NL, Williams JI, Yoshida KK, Bombardier C, Wright JG (1996) The context of measuring disability: Does it matter whether capability or performance is measured? *J Clin Epidemiol* **49**: 1097–1101.

Zwick EB, Leistritz L, Milleit B, et al. (2004) Classification of equinus in ambulatory children with cerebral palsy-discrimination between dynamic tightness and fixed contracture. *Gait Posture* **20**: 273–279.

Definitions and Measurements of Spasticity and Dystonia:

Pathways to Solve a Babylonian Confusion

Kaat Desloovere and Warren A Marks

KEY POINTS

- 'Spasticity' is the most popular, but also the most criticized term for the pathophysiological response to muscle stretch. The many definitions of 'spasticity' cause confusion and disagreement amongst researchers and clinicians and can potentially lead to misunderstandings and to wrong treatment decisions.
- Accurate and valid measurements of the pathophysiological neuromuscular response to muscle stretch is challenging, but crucial to properly select and fine-tune treatment interventions, to evaluate treatment effect and to ultimately optimize treatment modalities.
- The increased resistance against passive muscle involves neural and non-neural components, which need to be decomposed to ensure optimal patient-tailored treatment.
- Passive stretch and active movement elicit different expressions of what is clinically labeled as 'spasticity'.
- Dystonia is more prevalent in 'spastic' cerebral palsy than generally appreciated.
- Measuring dystonia with comorbid spasticity is difficult.
- Dystonia plays a role in disrupting motor control.
- Current treatments for dystonia, especially in the context of cerebral palsy (CP) have limited efficacy.

OPPORTUNITIES

- The consensus-based conceptual framework of the pathophysiological neuromuscular responses to passive stretch provides guidance for terminology, definitions, and measurements and facilitates communication amongst clinicians and researchers.
- There is considerable potential in instrumented techniques to measure spasticity that provides greater reliability, validity, and precession of measurement compared to the clinical spasticity scales.
- The large variability in the pathological muscle activation observed during stretch can be reduced by categorizing stretch reflexes in different patterns, which may encourage treatment individualized treatment planning.

- Novel measurements may lead to newly described phenomena and enhanced knowledge on underlying pathophysiological mechanisms of the neuromuscular responses to passive stretch.
- Of available treatments for dystonia associated with cerebral palsy, trihexyphenidyl, intrathecal baclofen, and deep brain stimulation seem to offer the most benefit.

Regulation of muscle tone is crucial to achieving normal posture and movement. The intact neuromuscular system automatically modifies muscle tone when muscles are stretched (Bar-On et al. 2015). Many neuromotor disorders are characterized by altered muscle tone. Hypertonia, i.e. abnormally increased tension, is the most prevalent primary problem (Sanger et al. 2003; Bar-On et al. 2015). The exact pathophysiology of hypertonia is complex and only partially understood. Sanger et al. (2003) specified the different clinical features of hypertonia as 'spasticity', 'dystonia', and 'rigidity'. Recently, an international group of experts highlighted the challenge of finding a proper terminology, a valid definition, and a proper approach for measuring the observed clinical picture of 'spasticity'. The clinical picture was specified as 'the pathophysiological neuromuscular response to muscle stretch' (van den Noort et al. 2017). Indeed, many uncertainties remain to properly term and define this clinical phenomenon and to properly measure the phenomenon in muscles at rest as well as in activated muscles. Moreover, recent research suggests that cerebral palsy (CP) most frequently shows complex movement phenotypes, representing a mixed picture rather than isolated spasticity or dystonia (Lumsden et al. 2019). Many uncertainties need to be urgently clarified by future research to enhance the understanding of the fundamental underlying mechanisms, improve precision diagnosis and treatment at the patient-specific level, and thereby ensure optimal care in children with CP. In this chapter, the summary of the current knowledge and the related remaining challenges are discussed. The chapter is organized into three sections: (1) definition and conceptual framework of spasticity and dystonia, (2) spasticity and dystonia in CP, and (3) remaining diagnostic and management challenges to be tackled.

DEFINITION AND CONCEPTUAL FRAMEWORK OF SPASTICITY AND DYSTONIA

Definition of Spasticity and Dystonia

DEFINITION OF SPASTICITY

For many years, there has been debate regarding the proper terminology to be used for the pathophysiological neuromuscular response to muscle stretch, and regarding a proper definition of this clinical symptom (Alhusaini 2014; van den Noort et al. 2017). Much of this debate stems from the lack of consensus on what is understood by the observed symptom.

The most commonly used term for the pathophysiological neuromuscular response to muscle stretch is 'spasticity', and the most frequently cited definition is the one by Lance (1980). Lance defined 'spasticity' as 'a motor disorder characterized by a velocity-dependent increase in tonic stretch reflexes with exaggerated tendon jerks, resulting from hyperexcitability of the stretch reflex, as one component of the upper motor neuron syndrome' (1980). This definition, which covers the muscle response to passive movement, gained much popularity, probably because of the clear link with the presumed pathophysiological mechanism and because it refers to the symptom as one problem of the upper motor neuron syndrome (Bar-On et al. 2015; van den Noort et al. 2017). Yet, Lance's original definition also caused much confusion. Part of the confusion may have been triggered by the use of the words 'tonic stretch reflexes', which may be misleading. Lance seems to have used these words out of the common context (Gracies 2005). Indeed, the stretch reflex has a phasic and a tonic component (Gracies 2005). The phasic response is the initial peak of action potential, resulting from a rapid increase in muscle tension and which is related to the stretch velocity, while the tonic response is a later low-frequency muscle firing, which is related to the amount of stretch, and which is observed throughout the entire stretch (Alhusaini 2014). To avoid confusion, Gracies simplified Lance's definition by referring to 'a velocity-dependent increase in reflexes to phasic stretch, in absence of volitional activity' (Gracies 2005). Part of the confusion may also be related to the fact that the term 'spasticity' is used to describe different phenomena. The brain injury that underlies CP causes a widespread disturbance in neural connectivity, with effects on widely dispersed neural circuits. Hence, the entire picture of the involved pathophysiological mechanisms induced by muscle stretch is much more complex than suggested by Lance's definition. The symptom involves several neural circuits that are more or less linked with different clinical observations, such as 'spastic catch', 'clonus', and 'spasms' (Sanger et al. 2003; Alhusaini 2014; van den Noort et al. 2017).

In 2003 an NIH sponsored interdisciplinary working group (Sanger et al. 2003) launched a new definition, which seemed, partly compatible with Lance's, but which remained closer to the clinical observations. They defined spasticity as 'hypertonia in which one or both of the following signs are present: (1) resistance to externally imposed movement that increases with increasing speed of stretch and (2) resistance to externally imposed movement that rises rapidly above a threshold speed or joint angle' (Sanger et al. 2003). This definition described 'spasticity' as one clinical feature of hypertonia in children (next to 'dystonia' and 'rigidity'). The definitions by Lance and by Sanger et al. seem to complement each other (van den Noort et al. 2017). Yet, another multidisciplinary consortium, the SPASM (a European thematic network to develop standardized measures of spasticity), concluded that different clinical features in patients with upper motor neuron syndrome are commonly combined, and therefore 'spasticity' should be defined more broadly. They defined spasticity as: 'disordered sensorimotor control, resulting from an upper motor neuron lesion, presenting as intermittent or sustained involuntary activation of muscles' (Burridge et al. 2005). This broad definition seems to encompass all positive motor symptoms of the upper motor neuron syndrome (i.e. the muscle overactivity, as opposed to the negative symptoms that refer to impaired movement and motor control) (van den Noort et al. 2017). Also in daily clinical practice, the term 'spasticity' is commonly used rather broadly, including involuntary muscle activity and movements, and even alterations of elastic muscle properties, leading to reduced joint mobility (Lorentzen et al. 2018). These differences between definitions cause confusion and disagreement amongst researchers and clinicians and can potentially lead to misunderstandings and to wrong treatment decisions in clinical practice.

DEFINITION OF DYSTONIA

Dystonia is defined as a movement disorder in which involuntary sustained or intermittent muscle contractions cause twisting and repetitive movements, abnormal postures, or both (Sanger et al. 2003). While spasticity is mediated via the corticospinal pathways, dystonia is mediated via the basal ganglia, thalamus, and cerebellum. Conceptually, spasticity mediation is a direct two-way link from the sensorimotor cortex to the muscle via the spinal cord. Inhibitory input from the cortex serves to modulate the excitatory spinal cord efferent output. As such, spasticity is mostly binary – on or off. Spasticity is primarily mediated by the inhibitory neurotransmitter gamma aminobutyric acid in the spinal cord via the corticospinal pathways, thus limiting opportunities for centrally acting pharmacological amelioration. Dystonia is strongly associated with basal ganglia and thalamic lesions and associated connectivity pathways with the cerebellum and cortex. Movement is the result of the orderly sequential firing of neurons. Gait is one of the primary work products of movement. The basal ganglia circuitry, which is mediated by multiple neurotransmitters, maintains the balance between excitatory and inhibitory forces. Smooth movement requires the balance between multiple neurotransmitter systems offering more opportunities for intervention. The lack of balance results in the twisting, writhing, patterned movements we define as dystonia. More recently, dystonia has been recognized as a disorder of movement execution brought about by faulty somatosensory input in anticipation of a planned volitional movement and dependent (Hallett 2000). The final common pathway for movement is the action of acetylcholine at the neuromuscular junction, another largely poorly modulated on-off system.

Conceptual Framework of 'Spasticity'

The wide spectrum of spasticity definitions does not help the communication between clinicians and researchers and impedes the development of valid treatment algorithms. However, rather than promoting one definition above the other, or trying to achieve one overall agreement on the definition to be used, effort should be put in achieving consensus on a conceptual framework of the pathophysiological neuromuscular response to muscle stretch (van den Noort et al. 2017). The need for a clear diagnostic conceptual framework was recognized by an international group of experts, who contributed to a Delphi consensus study that defined an unambiguous terminology about involved concepts. The focus was on the identification of different mechanisms that give rise to involuntary muscle contractions resulting in increased resistance when stretching muscles at rest. The 37 experts who participated in the consensus meetings (in 2014 and 2015) were specialized in treating and/or assessing spasticity in clinical and/or research settings. The resulting conceptual framework enabled an unambiguous terminology to describe the phenomenon of pathophysiological neuromuscular response to passive muscle stretch. The participants thereby agreed that the term 'hyper-resistance' should be used, instead of 'spasticity', to refer to the observed clinical picture. This group also conceptualized the contributing components to hyper-resistance, i.e. the non-neural or tissue related contribution and the neural contribution to the resistance against stretch, the latter being related to the central nervous system (van den Noort et al. 2017). The framework allows us to discuss the varying terminology and the different perceived phenomena, which have been used in literature and in daily clinic, to describe the observed pathological response to muscle stretch. The non-neural contribution to hyper-resistance or tissue properties involves elasticity, viscosity, and shortening. The neural contributions to hyper-resistance can be decomposed in 'stretch hyperreflexia', which represents the 'velocity dependent involuntary' component and the 'involuntary background activation', which represents the 'non-velocity dependent' component (van den Noort et al. 2017). The popular term 'spasticity' is linked to stretch hyperreflexia, while the other popular term 'stiffness' is related to passive tissue contributions. Involuntary background activation involves postural reflexes, non-selective activation, tonic stretch reflexes, and fixed background activation (van den Noort et al. 2017). The final conceptual framework resulting from the consensus study is presented in Figure 4.1 (bold terms in part A).

This novel framework can facilitate communication between clinicians and researchers since it allows us to relate the many different terms that are used in literature to one of the components of the framework. Examples of the varying terms are 'reflex-mediated and non-reflex-mediated stiffness' (Lorentzen et al. 2010; Willerslev-Olsen et al. 2013; Alhusaini 2014; Geertsen et al. 2015), 'reflex and intrinsic stiffness' (Mirbagheri et al. 2001), 'passive muscle stiffness' (Willerslev-Olsen et al. 2013; Lynn Bar-On et al. 2014; Brandenburg et al. 2016; Van Der Krogt et al. 2016), 'mechanical muscle stiffness' (Theis, Korff, and Mohagheghi 2015), or other combinations of these terms, as well as terms that are more frequently used in other pathologies, such as 'spastic myopathy' in stroke (Baude, Nielsen, and Gracies 2019) and 'spastic dystonia' (Gracies 2005; Lorentzen et al. 2018). Some examples of such terms are indicated in Figure 4.1 (part B).

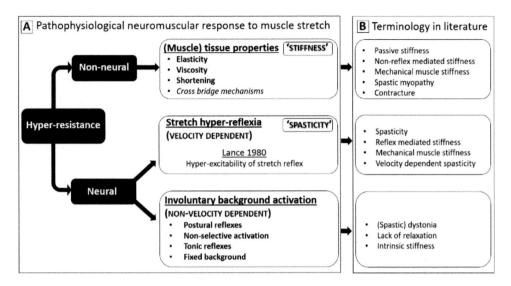

Figure 4.1 Part A: Conceptual framework of pathophysiological neuromuscular responses to passive stretch. Modified from van den Noort et al. 2017, with permission from Wiley; components written in italic were not included in the original framework. Part B: Terminology used in literature.

The components of the hyper-resistance in the framework can be measured, resulting in a variety of quantified outcome parameters (van den Noort et al. 2017). The challenges of measuring 'spasticity' in muscles will be discussed in the next section.

The framework developed by consensus amongst experts should not be considered as an endpoint since new information is constantly generated through research into pathophysiology and etiology of hyper-resistance. Novel measurements and insights in the pathophysiology lead to newly described phenomena that are proved to contribute to hyper-resistance, such as short-range stiffness (Groote, Allen, and Ting 2018). These novel concepts can also be linked to the components of the original framework (Fig. 4.1, cross bridge mechanisms in part A). The novel framework thus seems to provide a robust foundation for categorizing novel insights next to established knowledge.

Spasticity and Dystonia in CP

CP is the most common cause of childhood physical disability, with a prevalence of 2 to 3 per 1000 live births (Graham et al. 2016). This disorder is characterized primarily by neural deficits caused by a non-progressive lesion in the brain, and also by musculoskeletal problems that progress with age. Primary neuromotor deficits in CP are conceptualized as the direct result of brain anomalies and enclose mainly spasticity, weakness, and impaired muscle control. These problems influence growth and development of muscles and bones, resulting in changes in the muscle-tendon structure and in skeletal deformities (Gage et al. 2009). The primary and secondary motor deficits adversely affect typical development of functional activities such as walking. Several studies indicated that the primary neuromotor deficits, such as muscle spasticity and weakness, coexist in CP (Damiano et al. 2001; Øtensjø et al. 2004; Ross and Engsberg 2007; Kim and Park 2011). However, it still remains unclear how spasticity, weakness, and selective muscle control interact and how each impairment problem, or some combination, could eventually be the cause of functional deficits such as gait ([SCPE] Surveillance of cerebral palsy in Europe 2002). Because of the changes in the neural drive to muscles, and since muscles are one of the most plastic tissues in the body, children with CP experience significant alterations within the muscle. Macroscopically, there is evidence for reduced muscle volume, cross-sectional area, thickness, and belly length, with longer tendons and reduced muscle integrity in CP muscles compared to typically developing muscles (Barrett and Lichtwark 2010; Mockford and Caulton 2010; Theis, Korff, and Mohagheghi 2015; Theis, Mohagheghi, and Korff 2016). Microscopically, abnormally long muscle sarcomere lengths were observed, combined with fibre atrophy, variable fiber type predominance, and hypertrophic extracellular matrix of poor quality (Smith et al. 2012; De Bruin et al. 2014; Mathewson and Lieber 2015; Kinney et al. 2017; Lieber et al. 2017). Recent studies also indicated a reduced number of satellite cells, that may explain impaired muscle growth and poor responsiveness to training, such as strengthening (Smith, Chambers, and Lieber 2013; Dayanidhi and Lieber 2014; Dayanidhi et al. 2015; Kinney et al. 2017). The problem of altered muscle structure will be covered comprehensively in Chapter 8.

There is an overall agreement that 'spasticity' is the most frequently reported symptom in children with CP. However, the reported prevalence varies strongly between studies, from 62% up to 92% of the CP population ([SCPE] Surveillance of cerebral palsy in Europe 2002). This variability in prevalence may probably be explained by the confusing terminology and definitions that have been used. Yet, the majority of comprehensive cohort studies refer to a prevalence of 75% to 85% ([SCPE] Surveillance of cerebral palsy in Europe 2002; Lindén et al. 2019). While there is no doubt that 'spasticity' is frequently observed in children with CP, the relation between the spasticity and function remains confusing. Spasticity studies most frequently focus on muscles at rest. Yet, there is emerging evidence that passive stretch and active movement elicit different manifestations of what is clinically labeled as 'spasticity' (Lorentzen et al. 2010; Alhusaini 2014; Lorentzen et al. 2018). Part of the confusion on the role of spasticity during function may again be attributed to the lack of agreement on the terminology and definitions to be used. But the confusion seems also caused by the lack of an overall agreement in research, and especially in clinical practice, on how spasticity should be measured. Many challenges remain in the effort to 'quantify' spasticity into meaningful parameters that cover the entire picture. Therefore, the measurements of spasticity in muscles at rest and in activated muscles will be discussed in a separate section below.

CP can be often detected (suspected) as early as 3 months of age. Efforts are underway to improve education regarding early detection of CP. One important value of early detection is to improve the opportunity for early intervention (Novak et al. 2017). CP can be considered, at least in part, as a central nervous system driven neuromuscular disorder. Several studies showed that spasticity in children with CP increases during the first years of life. A recent register-based cohort study in Sweden (including 4162 children with CP), based on spasticity levels defined by the clinical Ashworth scale, concluded that the degree of spasticity increased in most children over the first 5 years of life (Lindén et al. 2019). Subsequently, spasticity decreased in 65% of the children until 15 years of age (which was the endpoint of the cohort study). Yet, such large cohort studies on the development of spasticity are rare. There is a need for more longitudinal studies, and for extension and optimization of databases and registries, which can give valuable information on the onset and development of spasticity, to support long-term treatment planning and to provide proper control data for intervention studies on spasticity reduction treatment (Lindén et al. 2019).

The degree and contribution of dystonia in CP has been historically underestimated. In a survey of young people with CP in Europe, both spasticity and dystonia were identified by scoring on the hypertonia assessment tool in more than 80% of patients with CP; 60% or more of each were rated as significant. Isolated spasticity or dystonia was seen in only 17 and 6% of patients, respectively (Lumsden et al. 2019). Quantifying the relative contributions of spasticity and dystonia has been difficult (Gordon et al. 2006). In spastic CP, comorbid dystonia is common and seems to be the predominant movement abnormality in the upper extremities, whereas spasticity dominates in the lower extremities, at least in ambulatory patients in the Gross Motor Function Classification Scale (GMFCS) levels I and II. The coexistence of dystonia in spastic CP increases with the GMFCS level (Palisano et al. 2008). Especially in children with bilateral involvement, the degree of dystonia increases with increasing level of ambulatory dysfunction. The distribution of spasticity and dystonia seems to be inversely related to predominantly spasticity in lower extremities and dystonia in the upper extremities. In ambulatory patients with bilateral CP in GMFCS levels I and II, the dystonic component is minimal if present at all. This explains in large part their good response to selective dorsal rhizotomy, which reduces spasticity by specifically targeting the dorsal rootlets of the nerves and seems to be negatively affected by dystonia and poor selective motor control seen with higher levels of disability. The goal of ambulation in patients with bilateral CP in GMFCS level III is less consistent. Even with aggressive spasticity management, ambulation is not expected in patients in GMFCS levels IV and V.

The coexistence of dystonia in spastic CP has an impact on gait, mobility, and the potential interventions. This is reflected in the concomitant loss of selective motor control. Selective motor control is 'impaired ability to isolate the activation of muscles in a selected pattern, in response to demands of a voluntary posture or movement' (Sanger et al. 2006). The 'selective control assessment of the lower extremity' has been utilized as a reliable measure of lower extremity selective motor control in children with spastic CP (Fowler et al. 2009). Selective motor control seems to be more reflective of dystonia than spasticity (Zhou et al. 2019). In developing treatment plans, it seems important to look at the various components involved in selective motor control. This measure has been most widely applied in the evaluation of gait in CP. Less is known about the use of selective control assessment of the lower in other disorders of motor tone and, in particular, primarily or purely dystonic disorders. It was not included in a previous review of rating scales for dystonia (Albanese et al. 2013). In their recent study in selective motor control, Zhou et al. highlighted the need for the importance of evaluating treatments targeted specifically at improving impaired selective motor control (2019). The problems of selective motor control will be covered in more detail in Chapter 6.

The negative effects of uncontrolled hypertonia are cumulative over time, resulting in progressive neuromuscular deformity and physiological stress. Direct physical consequences include skeletal deformities, fractures, and other injuries often related to osteopenia, skin breakdown, scars (surgical and injury related), and pain and discomfort (from both disease and treatment). There are associated physiological consequences including pain, malnutrition, insomnia, respiratory embarrassment, cardiac dysfunction, and premature death. Furthermore, there are negative psychosocial effects on the individual (loss of independence and autonomy) family and caregivers such as social isolation, family discord (divorce), financial hardship, and forgotten siblings. Finally, there are economic impacts to be considered beyond just the direct medical costs. There is the loss of productivity for the individual, as well as family caregivers, and there is a risk of injury. Long-term care is expensive and often borne by the state or federal health systems. Somewhat analogous to other neuromuscular disorders where weakness is the predominant feature, the progression of musculoskeletal deformity also corresponds to loss of ambulation. This underscores the need for better treatments for the motor symptoms of CP.

Conclusion: The Babylonian Confusion on Spasticity and Dystonia

'Spasticity' is probably the most popular, but also most criticized term for the pathophysiological neuromuscular response to muscle stretch. This term should be used with care and should always be accompanied by a definition that specifies the envisioned scope. There seems an increasing consensus that the term 'spasticity' only refers to the neural component of the clinical symptom, favoring, but also categorizing the original narrow definition by Lance (1980). Broader definitions should be linked with broader terms, encompassing different contributing components to the resistance against muscle stretch. A first step to solve the Babylonian confusion is to unambiguously phrase each phenomenon that is being observed and/or investigated, and to avoid using terms out of the scope that they are meant for, as well as to avoid introducing new terms without widespread consensus.

The recent consensus-based framework for conceptualizing the pathophysiological neuromuscular response to passive muscle stretch considers concepts implicit rather than explicit (van den Noort et al. 2017), thereby avoiding 'competition' between terms and definitions. This may be considered as another major step to solve the Babylonian confusion on 'spasticity'. The consensus-based concept 'hyper-resistance' that is suggested to avoid confusion still needs to be embraced by clinicians and researchers in the field who tend to stick to the familiar term 'spasticity'. The framework confirms and emphasizes the need to distinguish non-neural from neural contributions to hyper-resistance and provides a clear structure on how different mechanisms influence the observed phenomenon. Communication can become more effective by linking the many terms that are used in clinical practice and in literature to the different concepts of this framework. This also counts for the novel pathophysiological mechanisms that are continuously being investigated, potentially resulting in new contributing components within the framework.

The study on the definitions and terminology used in this field also highlights that used terms seem to be pathology-specific. For example, clinical experts in CP and in stroke tend to use another language to describe similar phenomena. A consensus and framework on terminology and definitions that are valid for different neuromotor disorders, such as CP, stroke, traumatic brain injury, and multiple sclerosis, will encourage clinicians and researchers to use the same language in daily practice and can facilitate knowledge transfer between experts. Collaborations among different clinical fields can thereby be fostered, to further disentangle the Babylonian confusion.

Future research is needed toward describing the longitudinal development of the hyper-resistance against passive stretch from the earliest infancy throughout childhood, to identify critical periods for treatment. Due to the lack of longitudinal studies, it remains unclear whether current treatment, for example botulinum neurotoxin A injections, are beneficial or detrimental in the long-term.

Finally, a remaining difficulty is the definition of the prevalence and the relevance of the coexistence of spasticity and dystonia. Mixed hypertonia, with components of spasticity and dystonia, is likely to be found in a much higher number of children with CP than originally thought. Yet, proper definitions of spasticity and dystonia are needed to identify the contribution of each to functional movements on a patient-specific level.

MEASUREMENT OF SPASTICITY AND DYSTONIA

To avoid confusion and to follow the guidelines of the previously introduced European consensus (van den Noort et al. 2017), the term 'hyper-resistance' will be preferred in the following sections, and the term 'spasticity' will only be used when specifically referring to the hyper-resistance component 'velocity dependent stretch hyperreflexia' (Lance 1980; van den Noort et al. 2017). The large number of patients affected, and the variety and complexity of treatment interventions emphasize the need for accurate measurement of hyper-resistance in order to define selection criteria for treatment interventions, to better delineate and optimize the treatment, and to evaluate the effect of the treatment procedures. In section II, first, the different approaches to evaluate hyper-resistance in muscles at rest are summarized and discussed, followed by a review and discussion on measurements of hyper-resistance in active muscles. In a separate section, the measurement of dystonia is also briefly discussed. These summaries and discussions are then used in section III, as a framework to highlight novel findings and remaining challenges.

Measurement of Hyper-Resistance in Muscles at Rest

CLINICAL SCALES FOR HYPER-RESISTANCE

Several clinical scales for hyper-resistance and related phenomena have been described. Thereby, the hyper-resistance is defined by sensing the resistance to stretching the muscle at rest, i.e. with the patient in a relaxed position. The most widely applied clinical method for the assessment of hyper-resistance is the Ashworth scale or its modified version (Bohannon and Smith 1987). In this scale, tone is graded according to the resistance perceived by the assessor during passive motion of the limb. Since these scales are based on ratings, they are prone to be subjective. With some exceptions (Meseguer-Henarejos et al. 2018), the reliability of these clinical assessments has repeatedly been questioned (Platz et al. 2005; Mutlu, Livanelioglu, and Gunel 2008). Also, their validity has been questioned (Pandyan et al. 1999; Biering-Sørensen, Nielsen, and Klinge 2006; Lorentzen et al. 2010; Bar-On et al. 2015), since the resistance felt is not solely due to the neural component of hyper-resistance but also due to non-neural components of resistance to muscle stretch. Moreover, the Ashworth scale does not address the velocity-dependent aspect of the phenomenon, as described by Lance (1980). The Tardieu scale (Tardieu, Shentoub, and DelarueE 1954) has been suggested as a more suitable alternative to the Ashworth scale for measuring hyper-resistance, as it assesses and compares the response of the muscle to passive movement at different speeds. However, previous studies (Fosang et al. 2003; Platz et al. 2005; Mutlu, Livanelioglu, and Gunel 2008) reported large variability in the magnitude of angular measurements and the difference between the slow and fast measures between sessions. Other phenomena that have been related to hyper-resistance, for example spasms and clonus, can also be rated by clinical scales (Platz et al. 2005). Clinical assessments of hyper-resistance are attractive for their simplicity of use. They have been successfully used to roughly grade children with CP, as input for large cohort studies (Lindén et al. 2019). However, the subjective character intrinsic to these methods may restrict reliability of measurements (Pandyan et al. 1999; Platz et al. 2005; Mutlu, Livanelioglu, and Gunel 2008). Furthermore, a clustering effect has been observed in the scores, with most patients being grouped in the middle grades (Bohannon and Smith 1987). Therefore, it is now widely acknowledged that more objective, quantitative, and robust measurements are required. Yet, it is surprising that these scales have remained the only standard in the clinic.

INSTRUMENTED ASSESSMENTS FOR HYPER-RESISTANCE

A variety of neurophysiological and biomechanical approaches to measuring hyper-resistance has been described, resulting in different parameters to quantify hyper-resistance.

Neurophysiological assessments

Neurophysiological tests have been developed to quantify exaggerated reflex responses and particularly to gain understanding in the pathophysiological mechanisms involved. Neurophysiological approaches investigate mainly the electrical responses of the motor control system upon a variety of stimuli and conditions. Commonly applied neurophysiological approaches are assessments of the Hoffmannn reflex, the tendon reflex, and the stretch reflex (Voerman, Gregoric, and Hermens 2005). The more fundamental neurophysiological studies significantly improved our insight into the underlying mechanisms of spasticity. However, the scope of the neurophysiological methods is relatively small because it provides information about a limited number of neural pathways that may cause spasticity (Burridge et al. 2005).

Biomechanical assessments

Biomechanical approaches study the behaviour of muscles, joints, and limb segments in response to movement. Approaches can be subdivided into three groups: (1) manual methods, (2) motor controlled methods, and (3) gravitational methods (Wood et al. 2005; Bar-On et al. 2014). The manual methods follow the basic approach of the common clinical practice, since passive manual stretches are applied (Pandyan et al. 2001; van den Noort, Scholtes, and Harlaar 2009; Bar-On et al. 2014). As a result, stretch reflexes are elicited. Joint angle and level of torque achieved during the pull can be measured, providing quantitative data. This is frequently combined with the collection of electromyography (EMG) data from the agonist and antagonist muscle group. It could be argued that the level of robustness for this method is small since the stretches are applied manually. Yet, for some of these measurement systems, the psycho-metrical properties were systematically evaluated and were found to be good (Bar-On et al. 2013; Bar-On et al. 2014; Bar-On et al. 2014; Schless et al. 2015). Moreover, this measurement approach is much appreciated (van den Noort et al. 2017) since it uses a relatively simple setup and could be constructed to be portable and simple to understand from a clinical perspective (Bar-On et al. 2013; Yamaguchi et al. 2018). The motor controlled methods (Lorentzen et al. 2010; De Vlugt et al. 2012) also measure response to passive movement, but in these methods, the joint rotation, speed and/or amplitude of movement are controlled by a motor, and is thus repeatable and accurate (Bar-On et al. 2015). Thereby, modelling of muscle behaviour during these well-controlled motions have been used to improve the understanding of the different components that contribute to the increased resistance to passive stretch. Unfortunately, these high-tech sophisticated methods are less appropriate for the clinical settings. Similar to the manual methods, angle characteristics are measured along with torque and EMG data. Different displacement waveforms, such as brisk and sinusoidal movements (Lee et al. 2004; Wood et al. 2005; Pandyan et al. 2006; Sloot et al. 2017), have been applied. The use of brisk stretches (Burridge et al. 2005) are more closely linked to the clinical Ashworth and Tardieu scales. It has also been suggested that the sinusoidal movements show similarities to functional movements, such as walking. Yet, the imposed movement profile is different between manual and motorized instrumented assessments of hyper-resistance, especially with respect to the applied accelerations (Sloot et al. 2017). At least at the ankle joint, the manually applied velocity profile matches more closely with the movement profile during gait (Sloot et al. 2017). Finally, gravitational methods involve lifting the limb under investigation against gravity to full extension and, when relaxed, releasing it, causing it to fall and swing freely. This approach has been most frequently used to study hyper-resistance at the level of the knee, where the lower leg is allowed to swing freely under the influence of gravity, while joint kinematics are recorded, often combined with EMG. It is commonly referred to as the (Wartenburg) pendulum test (Fowler, Nwigwe, and Ho 2000). The pendulum test is obviously challenging to be used for all joints.

Parameters that quantify hyper-resistance

When joint angles, torques, and EMG are recorded at different stretch velocities, the components of hyper-resistance described in the conceptual framework (Fig. 4.1) can be quantified. A complete overview of outcome parameters for hyper-resistance can be found in literature (van den Noort, Scholtes, and Harlaar 2009; Bar-On et al. 2014; Cenni et al. 2015; van den Noort et al. 2017). The direct outcome parameters for the neural component of hyper-resistance are related to the neurophysiological signal and include the amount of reflex activity measured by EMG (such as the averaged amplitude over a certain period), the timing of EMG onset, the stretch reflex velocity threshold, i.e. the joint velocity at which EMG onset is first detected (or the estimated lengthening velocity at EMG onset), and the duration of EMG activity. Thereby, the main focus is on the difference in EMG data between fast and slow stretches. The outcome parameters for the non-neural component are commonly defined from stretches at slow velocity and include the joint range of motion and the torque (at specific joint angles or the linear relation between joint angle and torque). Instrumented assessments also allow us to quantify the angle of catch (van den Noort, Scholtes, and Harlaar 2009; Wu et al. 2010; Bar-On et al. 2012) and its intensity

(Bar-On et al. 2012) by integrating biomechanical and neurophysiological data during fast stretch. The concrete decomposition of the neural and non-neural components of measured resistance (i.e. torque) can be achieved by comparing outcome parameters defined at different stretch velocities. Yet, this decomposition remains quite challenging, requiring a modelling approach (see separate section below). While many promising instrumented measurement setups for hyper-resistance have been introduced in literature to define the different outcome parameters, only a minority of these methods have been properly tested for reliability and validity (Bar-On et al. 2013; Bar-On et al. 2014; Bar-On et al. 2014; Schless et al. 2015).

Conclusion

Several literature reviews on the measurement of hyper-resistance have been published (Johnson 2002; Wood et al. 2005; Flamand, Massa-Alarie, and Schneider 2013; Bar-On et al. 2014). Each of the reviews has a slightly different perspective on the measurement of hyper-resistance, but the authors appear to converge on the following points: (1) there is considerable potential in instrumented techniques that can provide greater reliability and precession of measurement compared to the clinical scales; (2) both biomechanical and EMG measures of the stretch response need to be studied simultaneously in one setup, since each of these measures in isolation do not enable a distinction to be made between non-neural and neural factors contributing to the overall resistance to passive stretch, different methods of measurement are required to quantify the different contributing components; (3) because of the complex nature of hyper-resistance, an assessment may need to generate more than one 'value' of hyper-resistance; (4) while there is clearly a place for highly technical and sophisticated motor-driven measures to provide more insight in the underlying mechanisms of the hyper-resistance in a research laboratory setting, such methods are unlikely to be clinically useful. The discrepancy between the measurements for hyper-resistance that are now used in clinical practice and those that are used in research laboratories is striking. The problem is that most of the instrumented methods described above demand expertise and technology that may be too demanding for routine clinical use. Moreover, these integrated measurement systems have been poorly tested in the clinical environment and are not commercially available. Hence, there is an urgent need for developing easy-to-use measurement systems that can support clinicians in clinical diagnosis and decision making, and for enhancing specific training in instrumented assessments for clinical experts in CP.

Measurement of Hyper-Resistance in Activated Muscles

The commonly applied evaluations during a routine physical exam only represent the evaluation of hyper-resistance in muscles at rest, which covers just one level of the International Classification of Functioning, Disability, and Health (ICF) model, i.e. 'body functions and structures' (WHO 2020). The ICF model is recommended as a framework to guide diagnostic description and treatment planning. Hence, the role of hyper-resistance on the other ICF levels should also be studied, in particular with respect to the activity level (van den Noort et al. 2017). Yet, so far, the majority of studies have focused solely on hyper-resistance in muscles at rest, and its role during active movement is not yet entirely clear. But, it is increasingly acknowledged that muscles at rest and active muscles elicit different manifestations of hyper-resistance (Alhusaini 2014; Lorentzen et al. 2016). Previous research in this field can be categorized into two domains: (1) the study of relations between features of hyper-resistance measured in muscles at rest and features of gait, and (2) the study of hyperactive stretch reflexes in muscles that are active in isolation and during gait.

RELATIONS BETWEEN HYPER-RESISTANCE AND GAIT

The ultimate goal of any treatment in CP is to improve function, such as gait. Many treatment modalities focus on impairment level, assuming that this will improve gait (Ross and Engsberg 2007; Kim and Park

2011). Hyper-resistance represents only one impairment, next to, for example, weakness and contractures. Therefore, improved insight into the interaction between hyper-resistance and gait may significantly impact the clinical decision-making process. However, different studies highlight the complex relationship between hyper-resistance and gait (Ross and Engsberg 2007; Van Der Krogt et al. 2010; Kim and Park 2011), leaving the interactions largely unclear. The inherent complexity of gait, the collinearity between different underlying impairments, and possibly nonlinear interactions between impairments and gait, might be responsible for these inconsistent findings.

Previous studies explored the relation of specific components of hyper-resistance defined in muscles at rest with features of gait. Studies that relied on clinical scales to classify hyper-resistance (McMulkin et al. 2000; Desloovere et al. 2006; Choi et al. 2018) reported overall weak linear relations (correlations <0.40) between hyper-resistance grades and gait features. Studies that used instrumented assessments to quantify hyper-resistance and explore its association with gait features reported conflicting results. For example, correlations between stretch reflex thresholds defined by instrumented assessments in muscles at rest and joint angular velocities defined during gait varied from weak to strong (Ada et al. 1998; Tuzson, Granata, and Abel 2003; Damiano et al. 2006; Marsden et al. 2012; Bar-On et al. 2014; Willerslev-Olsen et al. 2014). It has become clear that, despite a series of studies in literature, there remains confusion on the relation between hyper-resistance measured in muscles at rest and features of gait in children with CP.

Some previous studies (van der Krogt et al. 2009; Van Campenhout et al. 2014) searched for 'markers of spasticity' during gait. These studies hypothesized that signs of hyperreflexia during gait can be highlighted by increasing walking velocity, thereby enhancing the velocity-dependent nature of the neural component of hyper-resistance. Since walking speed alters gait in CP as well as in typically developing children (Stansfield et al. 2001; van der Linden et al. 2002; Schwartz, Rozumalski, and Trost 2008), indirect insight into the effect of hyperreflexia on gait can be achieved by studying the differences in the effect of increased walking velocity on gait in CP and typically developing children. Only a limited number of 'markers of spasticity' were detected (Van Campenhout et al. 2014). These were the speed-related changes in kinematic, kinetic, and EMG features in children with CP, that were not observed in typically developing children. These markers were mainly extracted from muscle-length and EMG data, more often from the gastrocnemius than from the hamstrings.

Finally, some research groups explored the relationship between muscle lengthening velocity and muscle activity during specific phases of the gait cycle. This approach was introduced more than 30 years ago by Crenna (1998), who described altered relations between muscle lengthening velocity and EMG during gait in children with CP compared to typically developing children, which were found to be muscle-specific, i.e. differences between the gastrocnemius and the hamstrings. Later studies (Lamontagne, Malouin, and Richards 2001; Van Der Krogt et al. 2010) only partly confirmed these initial findings and indicated much heterogeneity within and between patients.

Measurement of Dystonia

Taking into account that dystonia is assumed to be more prevalent in spastic CP than generally accepted, sensitive, reliable, and clinically accessible tools that have the capacity to separately define the level of spasticity and dystonia in each child with CP are urgently needed.

CLINICAL SCALES FOR DYSTONIA

Dystonia in childhood can be evaluated by means of different clinical dystonia scales, such as the Burke-Fahn-Marsden dystonia rating movement scale (Burke et al. 1985), the unified dystonia rating scale (Comella et al. 2003), and the Barry-Albright dystonia scale (Barry, VanSwearingen, and Albright 1999).

The Burke-Fahn-Marsden dystonia rating movement scale and the Unified Dystonia Rating Scale were developed to assess primary dystonia. The Barry-Albright dystonia scale was created by a modification of the Burke-Fahn-Marsden dystonia rating movement scale, to develop a specific measure for secondary dystonia. While good to excellent interrater, intrarater, test–retest reliability, and internal consistency were found, several intervention studies questioned the sensitivity of the Barry-Albright dystonia scale (Butler and Campbell 2000; Holloway et al. 2006; Rice and Waugh 2009; Vidailhet et al. 2009; Monbaliu et al. 2010; Marks et al. 2011). Since dystonia and choreoathetosis occur concurrently in dyskinetic CP (Christine et al. 2007; Krägeloh-Mann and Cans, 2009), the dyskinesia impairment scale was recently developed to facilitate separate assessments for dystonia and choreoathetosis (Monbaliu et al. 2012). This scale was found to be reliable to assess dystonia and choreoathetosis in dyskinetic CP. Yet, the reliability of the dystonia subscale was found to be lower than the choreoathetosis subscale (Vanmechelen et al. 2020).

Discrimination between dystonia and spasticity is challenging (Himmelmann et al. 2009). Therefore, the hypertonia assessment tool (Jethwa et al. 2010) has been designed to differentiate between the three different types of hypertonia (spasticity, dystonia, and rigidity). The scale was found to be reliable and valid to identify spasticity and the absence of rigidity and shows moderate reliability for dystonia.

INSTRUMENTED ASSESSMENTS FOR DYSTONIA

Next to the use of clinical dystonia scales, quantitative motion analysis may potentially be used to measure dystonia (Pavone, Burton, and Gaebler-Spira 2013). Recently, a systematic literature review investigated the availability of instrumented assessments to measure motor problems at all levels of the ICF model, and described a series of useful instruments and technologies (Haberfehlner et al. 2020). These techniques most frequently involved 3D motion capture and surface EMG, especially for upper extremity, and assessed voluntary movement expressed as spatiotemporal and kinematic features and involuntary movement as overflow of muscle activity. Yet the psychometric properties of these techniques and methods have rarely been defined. For example, the kinematic dystonia measurement was introduced to measure dystonia overflow movement that is not required for a task. While this method was found to be reliable (Kawamura, Klejman, and Fehlings 2012), it only measures one aspect of dystonia, and the measure is expected to show overlap with choreoathetosis (Vanmechelen et al. 2019). For upper limb motion, Gordon et al. objectively differentiated spasticity from dystonia based on overflow movements of the contralateral arm (2006), while Butler and Rose used a pediatric upper limb motion index based on joint kinematics to reflect upper limb pathology and a set of spatial-temporal values to distinct a spastic and dyskinetic movement disorder using regression analysis (2012). Future research is needed towards improved insights in lower and upper limb kinematic patterns of dystonia (Haberfehlner et al. 2020).

REMAINING CHALLENGES TO BE TACKLED

The Challenge to Decompose Neural and Non-Neural Components of Hyper-Resistance

The hyper-resistance graded through clinical scales includes the neural as well as non-neural components. Also, when using instrumented measurements while stretching the muscle at high velocity, both the neural and non-neural components are reflected in the outcome parameter torque. Yet, at stretch velocities below the threshold of the stretch reflex, the measured resistance is solely caused by the non-neural soft-tissue properties, involving elastic properties of the muscle, connective tissue, tendon, and joints. This non-neural component has previously also been labeled as 'passive stiffness' (Willerslev-Olsen et al. 2013; Bar-On et al. 2014; Brandenburg et al. 2016; Van Der Krogt et al. 2016) or 'non-reflex mediated stiffness' (Voerman,

Gregoric and Hermens 2005; Lorentzen et al. 2016). When muscle stretches are performed at a velocity that exceeds the spastic threshold velocity, a stretch response will be evoked, adding a neural contribution to the measured torque. This neural component has previously often been labeled as the 'velocity-dependent spasticity' (Lance 1980; Sanger et al. 2003), or 'reflex-mediated stiffness' (Lorentzen et al. 2010 and 2016; Vlugt et al. 2010; Willerslev-Olsen et al. 2013; Alhusaini 2014; Geertsen et al. 2015). Yet, the concrete differentiation between the non-neural and neural components requires a modelling approach. Bar-On et al. (2015) recently discussed different modelling approaches to decompose both components. They concluded that several torque decomposition models had been developed, but only a few have been applied in children with CP. While some of these models quantified only the non-neural components of hyper-resistance, i.e. elasticity (Harlaar et al. 2000) and viscosity (Meyer, McCulloch, and Lieber 2011), more sophisticated algorithms additionally modelled the neural contribution to hyper-resistance (Chung et al. 2008; Vlugt et al. 2010; de Gooijer-van de Groep et al. 2013). With one exception (Bar-On et al. 2014), the decomposition models have only been validated on data collected by motor-driven systems, that allow optimal control of the applied displacement and torque. One research group extracted the neural component based on measurements from the manually controlled instrumented assessments (Bar-On et al. 2014). Thereby, a simple model that describes stiffness and viscosity in healthy muscle was approximated from the algorithms introduced by de Vlugt et al. (2010) The parameter to estimate the neural component was found to be repeatable between assessments and to distinguish between CP and typically developing muscles. Additionally, unlike the torque-related parameters that contain both neural and non-neural components, the value of this novel parameter was found to decrease after botulinum neurotoxin A injections. Unfortunately, this simplified method cannot be used to estimate the amount of elasticity and viscosity. In conclusion, it remains challenging to differentiate the neural and non-neural components of hyper-resistance in a clinical environment. Moreover, the contributing factors to the non-neural components also need to be further explored. The existing models for torque decomposition rely on many assumptions, and the content validity of the decomposed components is not yet sufficiently clear. This can most likely be achieved by combining instrumented hyper-resistance assessments with muscle imaging (Bar-On et al. 2018; Kalkman et al. 2018) and modelling work. Recently, instrumented measurements of hyper-resistance have been successfully combined with dynamic ultrasound measures tracking the muscle-tendon junction. These integrated measures can investigate the muscle and tendon lengthening during passive joint movements at different velocities and explore their interdependency with the elicited hyperactive stretch reflexes (Kalkman et al. 2016; Bar-On et al. 2018). This remains an important challenge for future research, which may have a crucial impact on the clinical decision making. A robust and validated differentiation between the neural and non-neural components of hyper-resistance remains a critical need for greater precision in diagnosis and treatment at the level of the individual with CP.

The Challenge of Measuring and Understanding the Component of Involuntary Background Activation

The neural contributions of hyper-resistance (Fig. 4.1) are subdivided into stretch hyperreflexia and involuntary background activation. Postural reflexes, non-selective activation, tonic reflexes, and fixed background tone have been specified as potential components of the involuntary background activation. This non-velocity dependent background activation is sometimes observed during stretches at very low velocity and might also be influenced by other phenomena (Lin 2004). For example, it may refer to the coexistence of dystonia in spastic CP. This hypothesis can be related to the concept of 'spastic dystonia', that has been defined as a 'tonic, chronic, involuntary muscle contraction in absence of any stretch or any voluntary command' (Pandyan et al. 2006; Lorentzen et al. 2018). There are a number of possible pathophysiological mechanisms that may be involved in the development of spastic dystonia, which have been recently discussed (Lorentzen et al. 2018). As previously highlighted, the measurement of dystonia in combination with spasticity remains a challenge for future research.

On the other hand, patients may face difficulties to fully relax during the instrumented assessments, and may thereby assist or prevent an imposed movement, or experience pain during the movement, challenging the discrimination of muscular activity from the pathological involuntary background activation. In fact, trials in instrumented assessments that include muscle activity that cannot be explained are frequently classified as noise and therefore excluded for further analyses (Bar-On et al. 2013; Schless et al. 2015; Lorentzen et al. 2016). Yet, these data may include important information on the non-velocity dependent neural component of hyper-resistance. Future research is needed to improve our understanding of the underlying factors of background muscle activation and their role in the clinical decision-making process.

The Potential Contribution of Cross-Bridge Mechanisms

Recent research (De Groote et al. 2018) suggests that muscle short-range stiffness in the presence of increased background muscle activity may play an important role in the initial response to stretch. Muscle short-range stiffness leads to a sharp increase in muscle force upon stretch that is proportional to the isometric muscle force before the stretch and hence increases with background muscle activity (Campbell and Moss 2002). This increase in force is due to short-range stiffness is dependent on movement history, with stiffness increasing when the muscle is held at a constant length (Campbell and Moss 2002). In addition, animal experiments have shown that history-dependent muscle force is encoded in muscle spindles (Blum et al. 2017). When a muscle is repeatedly stretched after being held at a constant length, the increase in force and the muscle spindle firing rate is found to be higher on the first stretch than on the following stretches. Model-based simulations suggested that hyper-resistance to imposed stretches results from the interaction between force encoding in muscle spindles and muscle dynamics (De Groote et al. 2018). In particular, modeling short-range stiffness and its interaction with background muscle activity was crucial to explain the observed movement during passive stretches in individuals with different levels of hyper-resistance. A follow-up experimental study manipulated short-range stiffness by making small oscillatory joint movements before the stretch (Willaert et al. 2020). Reducing short-range stiffness through premovement indeed reduced hyper-resistance to stretch, providing experimental evidence for the contribution of short-range stiffness to the response to imposed stretches in patients with hyper-resistance. Further research is needed to elucidate the interaction between history-dependent muscle dynamics that depends on background activity and stretch hyperreflexia.

The Role of Classifying Stretch Reflex Patterns

A large variability in the muscle activation patterns during muscle stretch has been observed in children with CP (Lebiedowska and Fisk 2009; Bar-On et al. 2014). Previous research suggested that reflex activity can be both length and velocity dependent (Fleuren, Nederhand, and Hermens 2006; Pandyan et al. 2006; Lebiedowska and Fisk 2009; Bar-On, Aertbeliën, Molenaers, and Desloovere 2014). Hence, stretch reflexes may be categorized based on the stretch reflex thresholds. Using an instrumented assessment of hyper-resistance to evaluate lower limb muscles in children with CP, Bar-On et al. (2014) defined different patterns of stretch-reflex muscle activation, i.e. those that reacted more to a change in velocity, and those that reacted more to a change in length. These muscle activation patterns were found to be muscle-specific since earlier stretch reflex thresholds and less-velocity dependent activation was observed in the hamstrings and adductor muscles when compared to the gastrocnemius and rectus femoris. The description of different stretch reflex patterns suggests new pathways for research. The underlying pathophysiological mechanisms of different stretch reflex patterns remain to be explored, and future studies should especially investigate whether muscles with different patterns react differently to treatment. Considering the existence of length dependent patterns, standardized positions for assessments of hyper-resistance are very important, especially when studying biarticular muscles, where the position of both joints are defining the muscle length. With respect to the velocity-dependent patterns, applied passive motions should also be performed at standardized velocities, especially for manual instrumented assessments. With some exceptions (van den Noort, Scholtes, and Harlaar 2009; Schless et al. 2015; Yamaguchi et al. 2018), the descriptions of standardized postures and movements have been incomplete or even lacking in previous studies. For future research, improved standardization of the measurements will facilitate data comparison and eventually encourage data-pooling between centers. Finally, a recent study (Sloot et al. 2017) suggested that especially differences in acceleration, rather than velocity, may account for the different muscle responses, which may suggest acceleration, rather than velocity-dependency of the stretch reflex. This novel paradigm needs to be further investigated.

Interactions Between the Components of Hyper-Resistance

The neural and non-neural components of hyper-resistance are expected to interact. Since cross-bridge stiffness (non-neural property) is history-dependent (because it increases proportional with baseline tonic muscle activity [Campbell and Moss 2002]), the involuntary background activation, which is a neural property, may influence the observed hyper-resistance. It is also likely that stretch reflex hypersensitivity (neural components) may occur in conjunction with length changes (non-neural component) (Alhusaini 2014). In contracted muscles, increased stretch-induced stimulation of spindles is expected, since the stretching force is more efficiently transmitted to the spindles in less extensible muscles (Gracies 2005). Also, within the neural components of hyper-resistance, interaction is anticipated. For example, background activation may interact with the stretch responses. When patients are not fully relaxed, cross-bridge formation between myosin and actin filaments will increase the resistance against stretch (Sinkjaer et al. 1993). This component has been labelled as 'intrinsic stiffness', next to the 'passive stiffness' and 'reflex-mediated stiffness'. It is challenging to distinguish these three components (Nielsen 2004). So far, the interactions between the components of hyper-resistance have been under-studied, and many hypotheses still need to be tested.

The Mystery of 'Spasticity' During Function

It remains challenging to define how different components of hyper-resistance influence function. On one hand, conventional gait analysis data, especially when walking at higher speed, seem to include some markers of hyper-resistance. A frequently observed example is the peak premature EMG activity in the plantar flexors in early stance when the muscles are rapidly stretched after toe contact (Burridge et al. 2001; Van Campenhout et al. 2014). On the other hand, several studies (Willerslev-Olsen et al. 2014; Willerslev-olsen, et al. 2018) questioned the role of the neural component of hyper-resistance in active conditions. These studies concluded that the neural component of hyper-resistance has a relatively minor contribution to pathological movement patterns of patients with neuromotor disorders, such as in CP or stroke. The non-neural components are suggested to play the more dominant role (Dietz and Sinkjaer 2007; Alhusaini 2014). Therefore, functional problems may be falsely attributed to stretch hyperreflexia, leading to inappropriate treatment planning. However, so far, most studies of reflexes during gait have been performed on adults, and all studies investigated only the plantar flexors. Studies in children with CP are rare, and due to the complex measurement setup, rather mildly involved patients have been enrolled in the study samples. Finally, the results of these studies are characterized by a large variability. Therefore, more research is needed to be able to generalize the findings and make strong concluding statements on treatment paradigms.

The Challenge of Treating Dystonia with Comorbid Spasticity

Uncontrolled hypertonia produces changes in the muscle, which may result in other impairments, such as weakness. The mechanisms of altered muscle growth are the topic of Chapter 8. Of importance here, however, is that treatments directed at central motor control are most effective before the permanent muscle pathology has been established. In an early study of deep brain stimulation in patients with mixed tone CP, there was a better response to therapy in younger patients who had less musculoskeletal contracture (Marks et al. 2011). Indeed, early management of dystonia is important, as the duration of dystonia before adequate intervention has a negative correlation with outcome in many disorders, including CP (Lumsden et al. 2013). This effect was partially reflected in a comparative study of deep brain stimulation in CP compared to Dyt-1 dystonia. Dystonia severity and duration of illness were both more severe in the CP population, thereby limiting the degree of functional gain (Marks et al. 2013). Earlier use of deep brain stimulation may provide better opportunity for early relief. Beyond the technical difficulties of implanting hardware into the underdeveloped brain, there may be an increased risk of complications, including the need for lead replacement surgery due to the increased time for head and neck growth that occurs before seven years of age.

Unilateral CP may be seen with white matter injury or, more commonly, with a stroke involving cortical gray and associated white matter fibers. In this case, there is often dystonia, which makes treatment of the corticospinal tract mediated spasticity less effective.

Pharmacological treatment of dystonia is complex. With the multiple neurotransmitter systems involved, most can be both up or down-regulated. Unfortunately, there is little solid evidence for the use of any of these medications in children, and in particular, in CP (Fehlings et al. 2018). The target neurotransmitters are widespread throughout the nervous system as well as many peripheral organs, especially the gastrointestinal system. Thus, the incidence of untoward effects is high, often limiting effectiveness. In addition, the long-term safety of these medications remains unknown. The best evidence of pharmacological efficacy is with anticholinergic medications. The doses needed for dystonia management are often well above typical doses in other disorders. Short term dose-related effects on memory and cognition have been well-recognized. More recently, a study in adult patients has raised concerns about increased risk of dementia with long-term use (Coupland et al. 2019).

Neither spasticity nor dystonia can be treated in isolation. At this time, our most aggressive and effective interventions for dystonia have been reserved for the most severely affected children meaning that end-organ changes in muscle have already occurred. Predictably measurable gains assessed by current rating scales are expectedly small. The ability to quantitate small but clinically important functional gains is also quite limited with the current assessment paradigms. This is a reflection of both the underlying severity of the brain injury and the delay in applying the available therapies. Cognitive impairment and muscle injury also limit the ability of the child to take functional advantage of tone reducing interventions. Hopefully, earlier recognition will lead to more aggressive application of tone management interventions. This is important, as we continue to strive for ways to remediate abnormalities of tone before irreversible damage to the end-organ muscle has occurred (Mathewson and Lieber 2015). Correcting the spasticity and dystonia after permanent structural musculoskeletal alterations will obviously limit the chances for functional improvement. Nonetheless, adequate tone management, even after musculoskeletal changes have occurred, is important in limiting progression of deformities and improving outcomes from orthopedic interventions.

Of course, the ultimate goal is prevention. Antenatal and early postnatal interventions reduce the prevalence and severity of CP by as much as 30% and up to 75% of children with CP are now ambulatory (Novak et al. 2020). How this is shifting the balance of hypertonia between spasticity and dystonia is less clear. One would reasonably anticipate that the relative spasticity/dystonia ratio would increase.

CONCLUSION

Hyper-resistance in children with CP is complex and heterogeneous in manifestations, making the clinical decision making and research into relevant treatment modalities difficult. Moreover, research on the different components contributing to hyper-resistance and their pathophysiological mechanisms is in a state of dynamic discovery, and new information is constantly generated through basic and clinically applied research. Yet, many aspects of the pathophysiology of hyper-resistance remains unclear. From the discussions on the definition and conceptual framework, as well as on the measurement of hyper-resistance, and their remaining challenges, critical knowledge gaps and potential pathways for future research are emerging, and a set of priority recommendations can be identified.

5-YEAR PRIORITIES

- Definitions and conceptual framework:
  - Accept and use unambiguously standardized concepts and terminology for hyper-resistance and avoid introducing new terms and definitions without widespread consensus amongst researchers and clinicians.
  - Integrate novel pathophysiological mechanisms that emerge from ongoing research within the consensus-based framework.
  - Describe the longitudinal development of the hyper-resistance from the earliest infancy throughout childhood, through optimizations of databases and registries.
- Measurements of hyper-resistance:
  - Accept the approach of instrumented assessment of hyper-resistance in muscles at rest as common practice for research and clinical practice.
  - Develop a set of reliable and valid outcome parameters for quantifying hyper-resistance.
  - Investigate the content validity of the non-neural components of hyper-resistance by combining instrumented hyper-resistance assessments with muscle imaging and modelling.
  - Improve the knowledge of the underlying factors of background muscle activation and on their role in the clinical decision-making process.
  - Investigate the contribution of short-range stiffness to hyper-resistance and its interaction with stretch hyperreflexia.
  - Enhance the understanding of the pathophysiological mechanisms of different stretch reflex patterns and investigate whether these patterns react differently to treatment.
  - Investigate to what extent differences in acceleration, rather than velocity, accounts for the different muscle responses during stretch.
  - Explore the interactions between the components of hyper-resistance.
  - Expand the study of reflexes during gait to larger samples of children with cerebral palsy, characterized by different severity of involvement and thereby focus on different lower limb muscles.

- Measurement of dystonia:
  - Develop a method that defines and quantifies the relative contribution and distribution of dystonia versus spasticity in CP, taking into account age-related motor development.
    - Subtraction technique to remove spasticity.
    - Challenging quantitative test to elicit dystonia.
    - Accelerometers and other wearables inertia measurement units for measuring daily function.
    - Inclusion of functional measures as part of testing, such as the time up and go test and the one minute walking test (Himuro et al. 2017).
    - 'Smarter assessments' such as more challenging assessments by means of motion capture systems.

FUTURE NEEDS

- Definitions and conceptual framework:
  - There is a need for one common language to describe hyper-resistance amongst clinicians and researchers, experts in different pathologies, and researchers with biomechanical and neurophysiological expertise.
  - There is a need to compare hyper-resistance in diverse patient populations. Comparison of outcomes across populations have been under-investigated.
  - Research on hyper-resistance should always consider the distinction between its non-neural and neural contributions, and the structure on how different mechanisms influence the observed phenomena.
- Measurements of hyper-resistance:
  - All instrumented setups to measure hyper-resistance in muscles at rest need to be properly tested for reliability and validity.
  - Improved standardization of the measurements is needed to facilitate data comparison and allow data-pooling between centers.
  - There is an urgent need for developing easy-to-use instrumented measurement systems that can support clinicians in clinical diagnosis and decision making.
  - Non-linear relationships between hyper-resistance defined in muscles at rest and features of gait should be explored.
  - We need integration of measures of hyper-resistance in muscles at rest with measures during function, such as gait analysis. This has been successfully achieved in healthy adults and in typically developing children (Willerslev-olsen et al. 2018), but this research is still scarce in patients with cerebral palsy.
  - We need an increasing academic focus on some understudied components of hyper-resistance, such as the background knowledge and the role of cross-bridge mechanisms.
  - There is a critical need for greater precision of hyper-resistance to allow treatment at the level of the individual with CP, in order to develop best-practice approaches for providing optimal care throughout childhood.
  - One potential source of variability insufficiently accounted for in existing research is the heterogeneity of hyper-resistance, which likely obscures interpretation of data on treatment responses from a mixed patient group. We need to categorize different patterns of hyper-resistance and improved approaches to quantify distinguished features of hypertonia. Especially, the overlap between hyper-resistance and dystonia needs to be further explored.
  - Training of cerebral palsy clinicians and investigators need to be enhanced.
  - Clinical practice and research need to keep pace when studying hyper-resistance.

- Measurement and treatment of dystonia combined with spasticity:
  - There is a need for an improved understanding of causal pathways.
    - Are the underlying pathways of dystonia in cerebral palsy the same as those in other dystonias, or does early brain injury influence the anatomic organization?
    - Would more aggressive earlier intervention for the treatment limit the negative neuromuscular and orthopedic consequences of dystonia?
  - With the knowledge that the duration of abnormal tone may be correlated with permanent changes in neuromuscular structure and bony alignment, there is a need to investigate how early interventions in the course of cerebral palsy can be developed and/or modified and how irreversible pathological changes in the muscle can be prevented.
  - More research is needed to determine the relative priority for treating spasticity or dystonia in a given patient. It remains unclear whether treating one necessarily exacerbates or unmasks the other.
  - With the limited response to pharmacological management in many patients with dystonia, future studies are needed to define whether neurosurgical interventions (selective dorsal rhizotomy, deep brain stimulation, intrathecal baclofen) should be considered earlier in childhood.
  - More research is needed to evaluate whether the current approach of 'tone than bones' is necessarily correct, or whether earlier orthopedic intervention in selected patients allow better response to tone management.

REFERENCES

(SCPE) Surveillance of cerebral palsy in Europe (2002) Prevalence and characteristics of children with cerebral palsy in Europe. *Developmental medicine and child neurology* **44**: 633–640.

Ada L, Vattanasilp W, O'Dwyer NJ, Crosbie J (1998) Does spasticity contribute to walking dysfunction after stroke? *Journal of neurology, neurosurgery, and psychiatry* **64**: 628–635.

Albanese A, Sorbo FD, Comella C et al. (2013) Dystonia rating scales: critique and recommendations. *Movement disorders: official journal of the Movement Disorder Society* **28**: 874–83.

Alhusaini AA (2014) Functional effects of neural impairments and subsequent adaptations, In: Shepherd RB editors, *Cerebral aplsy in infancy*. Sidney: Elsevier, pp 87–106.

Bar-On L, Aertbeliën E, Guy M et al. (2013) Comprehensive quantification of the spastic catch in children with cerebral palsy. *Research in developmental disabilities* **34**: 386–396.

Bar-On L, Aertbeliën E, Wambacq H et al. (2013) A clinical measurement to quantify spasticity in children with cerebral palsy by integration of multidimensional signals. *Gait and Posture* **38**: 141–147.

Bar-On L, Desloovere K, Molenaers G, Harlaar J, Kindt T, Aertbeliën E (2014) Identification of the neural component of torque during manually-applied spasticity assessments in children with cerebral palsy. *Gait and Posture* **40**: 346–351.

Bar-On L, Aertbeliën E, Molenaers G et al. (2014) Instrumented assessment of the effect of Botulinum Toxin-A in the medial hamstrings in children with cerebral palsy. *Gait and Posture* **39**: 17–22.

Bar-On L, Van Campenhout A, Desloovere K et al. (2014) Is an instrumented spasticity assessment an improvement over clinical spasticity scales in assessing and predicting the response to integrated botulinum toxin type A treatment in children with cerebral palsy? *Archives of Physical Medicine and Rehabilitation* **95**: 515–523.

Bar-On L, Aertbeliën E, Molenaers G, Dan B, Desloovere K (2014) Manually controlled instrumented spasticity assessments: A systematic review of psychometric properties. *Developmental Medicine and Child Neurology* **56**: 932–950.

Bar-On L, Aertbeliën E, Molenaers G, Desloovere K (2014) Muscle activation patterns when passively stretching spastic lower limb muscles of children with cerebral palsy. *PLoS ONE* **9**: e91759.

Bar-On L, Molenaers G, Aertbeliën E, Monari D, Feys H, Desloovere K (2014) The relation between spasticity and muscle behavior during the swing phase of gait in children with cerebral palsy. *Research in Developmental Disabilities* **35**: 3354–3364.

Bar-On L, Molenaers G, Aertbeliën E et al. (2015) Spasticity and its contribution to hypertonia in cerebral palsy. *BioMed Research International* **2015**: 317047.

Bar-On L, Kalkman BM, Cenni F et al. (2018) The relationship between medial gastrocnemius lengthening properties and stretch reflexes in cerebral palsy. *Frontiers in Pediatrics* **6**: 259.

Barrett RS, Lichtwark GA (2010) Gross muscle morphology and structure in spastic cerebral palsy: a systematic review. *Developmental Medicine and Child Neurology* **52**: 794–804.

Barry MJ, VanSwearingen JM, Albright AL (1999) Reliability and responsiveness of the Barry-Albright Dystonia Scale. *Developmental medicine and child neurology* **41**: 404–411.

Baude M, Nielsen JB, Gracies JM (2019) The neurophysiology of deforming spastic paresis: A revised taxonomy. *Annals of Physical and Rehabilitation Medicine* **62**: 426–430.

Biering-Sørensen F, Nielsen JB, Klinge K (2006) Spasticity-assessment: a review. *Spinal Cord* **44**: 708–722.

Blum KP, Lamotte D'Incamps B, Zytnicki D, Ting LH (2017) Force encoding in muscle spindles during stretch of passive muscle. *PLOS Computational Biology* **13**: e1005767.

Bohannon RW, Smith MB (1987) Inter rater reliability of a modified Ashworth Scale of muscle spasticity. *Phys Ther*, **67**: 206–207.

Brandenburg JE, Eby SF, Song P, Kingsley-Berg S, Bamlet W, Sieck GC, An KN (2016) Quantifying passive muscle stiffness in children with and without cerebral palsy using ultrasound shear wave elastography. *Developmental Medicine and Child Neurology*. **58**: 1288–1294.

de Bruin M, Smeulders MJ, Kreulen M, Huijing PA, Jaspers RT (2014) Intramuscular connective tissue differences in spastic and control muscle: A mechanical and histological study. *PLoS ONE* **9**: e101038.

Burke RE, Fahn S, Marsden CD, Bressman SB, Moskowitz C, Friedman J (1985) Validity and reliability of a rating scale for the primary torsion dystonias. *Neurology* **35**: 73–7.

Burridge JH, Wood DE, Taylor PN, McLellan DL (2001) Indices to describe different muscle activation patterns, identified during treadmill walking, in people with spastic drop-foot. *Medical Engineering and Physics* **23**: 427–434.

Burridge JH, Wood DE, Hermens HJ et al. (2005) Theoretical and methodological considerations in the measurement of spasticity. *Disability and rehabilitation* **27**: 69–80.

Butler C and Campbell S (2000) Evidence of the effects of intrathecal baclofen for spastic and dystonic cerebral palsy. AACPDM Treatment Outcomes Committee Review Panel. *Developmental medicine and child neurology* **42**: 634–645.

Butler EE and Rose J (2012) The pediatric upper limb motion index and a temporal-spatial logistic regression: quantitative analysis of upper limb movement disorders during the Reach and Grasp Cycle. *Journal of biomechanics* **45**: 945–951.

Campbell KS and Moss RL (2002) History-dependent mechanical properties of permeabilized rat soleus muscle fibers. *Biophysical journal* **82**: 929–943.

Van Campenhout A, Bar-On L, Aertbeliën E, Huenaerts C, Molenaers G, Desloovere K (2014) Can we unmask features of spasticity during gait in children with cerebral palsy by increasing their walking velocity? *Gait and Posture* **39**: 953–957.

Cenni F, Monari D, Schless SH, Bar-On L, Desloovere K (2015) Combining motion analysis and ultrasound to analyse muscles in children with cerebral palsy. *Gait & Posture* **42**: S2–S3.

Choi JY, Park ES, Park D, Rha DW (2018) Dynamic spasticity determines hamstring length and knee flexion angle during gait in children with spastic cerebral palsy. *Gait & Posture* **64**: 255–259.

Christine C, Dolk H, Platt MJ, Colver A, Prasauskiene A, Krägeloh-Mann I; SCPE Collaborative Group (2007) Recommendations from the SCPE collaborative group for defining and classifying cerebral palsy. *Dev Med Child Neurol Suppl* **109**: 35–38.

Chung SG, van Rey E, Bai Z, Rymer WZ, Roth EJ, Zhang LQ (2008) Separate Quantification of Reflex and Nonreflex Components of Spastic Hypertonia in Chronic Hemiparesis. *Archives of Physical Medicine and Rehabilitation* **89**: 700–710.

Comella CL, Leurgans S, Wuu J, Stebbins GT, Chmura T (2003) Rating scales for dystonia: A multicenter assessment. *Movement Disorders* **18**: 303–312.

Coupland CAC, Hill T, Dening T, Morriss R, Moore M, Hippisley-Cox J (2019) Anticholinergic Drug Exposure and the Risk of Dementia: A Nested Case-Control Study. *JAMA internal medicine* **179**: 1084–1093.

Crenna P (1998) Spasticity and "spastic" gait in children with cerebral palsy. *Neurosci Biobehav Rev* **22**: 571–578.

Damiano DL, Quinlivan J, Owen BF, Shaffrey M, Abel MF (2001) Spasticity versus strength in cerebral palsy: relationships among involuntary resistance, voluntary torque, and motor function. *European journal of neurology* **5**: 40–49.

Damiano DL, Laws E, Carmines DV, Abel MF (2006) Relationship of spasticity to knee angular velocity and motion during gait in cerebral palsy. *Gait and Posture* **23**: 1–8.

Dayanidhi S, Lieber RL (2014) Skeletal muscle satellite cells: Mediators of muscle growth during during development and implications for developmental disorders. *Muscle Nerve* **50**: 723–732.

Dayanidhi S, Dykstra PB, Lyubasyuk V, McKay BR, Chambers HG, Lieber RL (2015) Reduced satellite cell number in situ in muscular contractures from children with cerebral palsy. *Journal of Orthopaedic Research* **33**: 1039–1045.

Desloovere K, Molenaers G, Feys H, Huenaerts C, Callewaert B, Van de Walle P (2006) Do dynamic and static clinical measurements correlate with gait analysis parameters in children with cerebral palsy? *Gait and Posture* **24**: 302–313.

Dietz V and Sinkjaer T (2007) Spastic movement disorder: impaired reflex function and altered muscle mechanics. *Lancet Neurology* **6**: 725–733.

Fehlings D, Brown L, Harvey A et al. (2018) Pharmacological and neurosurgical interventions for managing dystonia in cerebral palsy: a systematic review. *Developmental Medicine & Child Neurology* **60**: 356–366.

Flamand VH, Massa-Alarie H and Schneider C (2013) Psychometric evidence of spasticity measurement tools in cerebral palsy children and adolescents: A systematic review. *Journal of Rehabilitation Medicine* **45**: 14–23.

Fleuren JF, Nederhand MJ, Hermens HJ (2006) Influence of Posture and Muscle Length on Stretch Reflex Activity in Poststroke Patients With Spasticity. *Archives of Physical Medicine and Rehabilitation* **87**: 981–988.

Fosang AL, Galea MP, McCoy AT, Reddihough DS, Story I (2003) Measures of muscle and joint performance in the lower limb of children with cerebral palsy. *Developmental medicine and child neurology* **45**: 664–670.

Fowler EG, Staudt LA, Greenberg MB, Oppenheim WL (2009) Selective Control Assessment of the Lower Extremity (SCALE): Development, validation, and interrater reliability of a clinical tool for patients with cerebral palsy. *Developmental Medicine and Child Neurology* **51**: 607–614.

Fowler EG, Nwigwe AI, Ho TW (2000) Sensitivity of the pendulum test for assessing spasticity in persons with cerebral palsy. *Dev Med Child Neurol* **42**: 182–189.

Gage JR, Schwartz MH, Koop SE, Novacheck TF (2009) *The Identification and Treatment of Gait Problems in Cerebral Palsy*. London: Mac Keith Press

Geertsen SS, Kirk H, Lorentzen J, Jorsal M, Johansson CB, Nielsen JB (2015) Impaired gait function in adults with cerebral palsy is associated with reduced rapid force generation and increased passive stiffness. *Clinical Neurophysiology* **126**: 2320–2329.

de Gooijer-van de Groep KL, de Vlugt E, de Groot JH et al. (2013) Differentiation between non-neural and neural contributors to ankle joint stiffness in cerebral palsy. *Journal of neuroengineering and rehabilitation*. **10**: 81.

Gordon LM, Keller JL, Stashinko EE, Hoon AH, Bastian AJ (2006) Can Spasticity and Dystonia Be Independently Measured in Cerebral Palsy? *Pediatric Neurology* **35**: 375–381.

Gracies JM (2005) Pathophysiology of spastic paresis. II: Emergence of muscle overactivity *Muscle and Nerve*, **31**: 552–571.

Graham HK, Rosenbaum P, Paneth N et al. (2016) Cerebral palsy. *Nat Rev Dis Primers* **2**: 15082.

De Groote F, Blum KP, Horslen BC, Ting LH (2018) Interaction between muscle tone, short-range stiffness and increased sensory feedback gains explains key kinematic features of the pendulum test in spastic cerebral palsy: A simulation study. *PloS one* **13**: e0205763.

De Groote F, Allen JL, Ting LH (2018) Contribution of muscle short-range stiffness to initial changes in joint kinetics and kinematics during perturbations to standing balance: A simulation study. *J Biomech* **55**: 71–77.

Haberfehlner H, Goudriaan M, Bonouvrié LA et al. (2020) Instrumented assessment of motor function in dyskinetic cerebral palsy: a systematic review. *J Neuroeng Rehabil* **17**: 39.

Hallett M (2000) Disorder of movement preparation in dystonia. *Brain: a journal of neurology* **123**: 1765–1766.

Harlaar J, Becher JG, Snijders CJ, Lankhorst GJ (2000) Passive stiffness characteristics of ankle plantar flexors in hemiplegia. *Clinical Biomechanics* **15**: 261–270.

Himmelmann K, McManus V, Hagberg G, Uvebrant P, Krägeloh-Mann I, Cans C; SCPE collaboration (2009) Dyskinetic cerebral palsy in Europe: trends in prevalence and severity. *Archives of Disease in Childhood* **94**: 921–926.

Himuro N, Abe H, Nishibu H, Seino T, Mori M (2017) Easy-to-use clinical measures of walking ability in children and adolescents with cerebral palsy: a systematic review. *Disability and Rehabilitation* **39**: 957–968.

Holloway KL, Baron MS, Brown R, Cifu DX, Carne W, Ramakrishnan V (2006) Deep Brain Stimulation for Dystonia: A Meta-Analysis. *Neuromodulation: Technology at the Neural Interface* **9**: 253–261.

Jethwa A, Mink J, Macarthur C, Knights S, Fehlings T, Fehlings D (2010) Development of the Hypertonia Assessment Tool (HAT): a discriminative tool for hypertonia in children. *Developmental medicine and child neurology* **52**: e83–e87.

Johnson GR (2002) Outcome measures of spasticity. *European journal of neurology: the official journal of the European Federation of Neurological Societies* **9**: 10–16.

Kalkman B, Bar-On L, Cenni F et al. (2016) Passive muscle and tendon properties during ankle joint rotation in children with cerebral palsy. *Gait & Posture.* **49**: 133–134.

Kalkman BM, Bar-On L, Cenni F et al. (2018) Medial gastrocnemius muscle stiffness cannot explain the increased ankle joint range of motion following passive stretching in children with cerebral palsy. *Exp Physiol* **103**: 350–357.

Kawamura A, Klejman S, Fehlings D (2012) Reliability and validity of the kinematic dystonia measure for children with upper extremity dystonia. *Journal of child neurology* **27**: 907–913.

Kim WH and Park EY (2011) Causal relation between spasticity, strength, gross motor function, and functional outcome in children with cerebral palsy: A path analysis. *Developmental Medicine and Child Neurology* **53**: 68–73.

Kinney MC, Dayanidhi S, Dykstra B, McCarthy JJ Perterson CA Lieber RL (2017) Reduced skeletal muscle satellite cell number alters muscle morphology after chronic stretch but allows limited serial sarcomere addition. *Muscle* **55**: 384–392.

Krägeloh-Mann I and Cans C (2009) Cerebral palsy update. *Brain and Development* **31**: 537–544.

van der Krogt MM, Doorenbosch CA, Becher JG, Harlaar J (2009) Walking speed modifies spasticity effects in gastrocnemius and soleus in cerebral palsy gait. *Clinical Biomechanics* **24**: 422–428.

van der Krogt MM, Doorenbosch CA, Becher JG, Harlaar J (2010) Dynamic spasticity of plantar flexor muscles in cerebral palsy gait. *Journal of Rehabilitation Medicine* **42**: 656–663.

van der Krogt MM, Bar-On L, Kindt T, Desloovere K, Harlaar J (2016) Neuro-musculoskeletal simulation of instrumented contracture and spasticity assessment in children with cerebral palsy. *Journal of NeuroEngineering and Rehabilitation* **13**: 64.

Lamontagne A, Malouin F, Richards CL (2001) Locomotor-specific measure of spasticity of plantarflexor muscles after stroke. *Archives of Physical Medicine and Rehabilitation* **82**: 1696–1704.

Lance J (1980) Spasticity: Disordered motor control. In Feldman RG, Young RR, Koella WP, editors, *Symposium synopsis*. Chicago: Medical Publisher, pp 485–495.

Lebiedowska MK and Fisk JR (2009) Knee resistance during passive stretch in patients with hypertonia. *Journal of Neuroscience Methods* **179**: 323–330.

Lee HM, Chen JJ, Ju MS, Lin CC, Poon PP (2004) Validation of portable muscle tone measurement device for quantifying velocity-dependent properties in elbow spasticity. *J Electromyogr Kinesiol* **14**: 577–589.

Lieber RL, Roberts TJ, Blemker SS, Lee SSM, Herzog W (2017) Skeletal muscle mechanics, energetics and plasticity. *Journal of NeuroEngineering and Rehabilitation* **14**: 108.

Lin J (2004) The assessment and management of hypertonus in cerebral palsy: a physiological atlas ("road map") In Scrutton D, Damiano D, Mayston M, editors, *Management of the Motor Disorders of Children with Cerebral Palsy Clinics in Developmental Medicine.* London: Mac Keith Press, pp. 85–104.

van der Linden ML, Kerr AM, Hazlewood ME, Hillman SJ, Robb JE (2002) Kinematic and kinetic gait characteristics of normal children walking at a range of clinically relevant speeds. *Journal of pediatric orthopedics* **22**: 800–806.

Lindén O, Hägglund G, Rodby-Bousquet E, Wagner P (2019) The development of spasticity with age in 4,162 children with cerebral palsy: a register-based prospective cohort study. *Acta Orthopaedica* **90**: 286–291.

Lorentzen J, Grey MJ, Crone C, Mazevet D, Biering-Sørensen F, Nielsen JB (2010) Distinguishing active from passive components of ankle plantar flexor stiffness in stroke, spinal cord injury and multiple sclerosis. *Clinical Neurophysiology* **121**: 1939–1951.

Lorentzen J, Kirk H, Fernandez-Lago H et al. (2016) Treadmill training with an incline reduces ankle joint stiffness and improves active range of movement during gait in adults with cerebral palsy. *Disabil Rehabil* **39**: 987–993

Lorentzen J, Willerslev-Olsen M, Hüche Larsen H et al. (2018) Feedforward neural control of toe walking in humans. *J Physiol* **11**: 2159–2172.

Lorentzen J, Pradines M, Gracies JM, Bo Nielsen J (2018) On Denny-Brown's 'spastic dystonia' – What is it and what causes it? *Clin Neurophysiol* **129**: 89–94.

Lumsden DE, Kaminska M, Gimeno H et al. (2013) Proportion of life lived with dystonia inversely correlates with response to pallidal deep brain stimulation in both primary and secondary childhood dystonia. *Dev med child* **55**: 567–574.

Lumsden DE, Crowe B, Basu A et al. (2019) Pharmacological management of abnormal tone and movement in cerebral palsy. *Archives of disease in childhood* **104**: 775–780.

Marks W, Bailey L, Reed M et al. (2013) Pallidal stimulation in children: comparison between cerebral palsy and DYT1 dystonia. *J Child Neurol* **28**: 840–848.

Marks WA, Honeycutt J, Acosta F Jr et al. (2011) Dystonia due to cerebral palsy responds to deep brain stimulation of the globus pallidus internus. *Movement Disorders* **26**: 1748–1751.

Marsden J, Ramdharry G, Stevenson V, Thompson A (2012) Muscle paresis and passive stiffness: Key determinants in limiting function in Hereditary and Sporadic Spastic Paraparesis. *Gait and Posture* **35**: 266–271.

Mathewson MA and Lieber RL (2015) Pathophysiology of Muscle Contractures in Cerebral Palsy. *Phys Med Rehabil Clin N Am* **26**: 57–67.

McMulkin ML, Gulliford JJ, Williamson RV, Ferguson RL (2000) Correlation of static to dynamic measures of lower extremity range of motion in cerebral palsy and control populations. *J Pediatr Orthop* **20**: 366–369.

Meseguer-Henarejos AB, Sánchez-Meca J, López-Pina JA, Carles-Hernández R (2018) Inter- and intra-rater reliability of the Modified Ashworth Scale: a systematic review and meta-analysis. *Eur J Phys Rehabil Med* **54**: 576–590.

Meyer GA, McCulloch AD and Lieber RL (2011) A Nonlinear Model of Passive Muscle Viscosity. *J Biomech Eng* **133**: 091007.

Mirbagheri MM, Barbeau H, Ladouceur M, Kearney RE (2001) Intrinsic and reflex stiffness in normal and spastic, spinal cord injured subjects. *Experimental Brain Research* **141**: 446–459.

Mockford M and Caulton JM (2010) The pathophysiological basis of weakness in children with cerebral palsy. *Pediatr Phys Ther* **22**: 222–233.

Monbaliu E, Ortibus E, Roelens F et al. (2010) Rating scales for dystonia in cerebral palsy: Reliability and validity. *Dev Med Child Neurol* **52**: 570–575.

Monbaliu E, Ortibus E, De Cat J et al. (2012) The Dyskinesia Impairment Scale: a new instrument to measure dystonia and choreoathetosis in dyskinetic cerebral palsy. *Dev Med Child Neurol* **54**: 278–283.

Mutlu A, Livanelioglu A, Gunel MK (2008) Reliability of Ashworth and Modified Ashworth scales in children with spastic cerebral palsy. *BMC musculoskeletal disorders* **9**: 44.

Nielsen JB (2004) Sensorimotor integration at spinal level as a basis for muscle coordination during voluntary movement in humans. *J Appl Physiol* **96**: 1961–1967.

Nielsen JB, Petersen NT, Crone C, Sinkjaer T (2005) Stretch Reflex Regulation in Healthy Subjects and Patients with Spasticity. *Neuromodulation* **8**: 49–57.

van den Noort JC, Bar-On L, Aertbeliën E et al. (2017) European consensus on the concepts and measurement of the pathophysiological neuromuscular responses to passive muscle stretch. *Eur J Neurol* **24**: 981–e38.

van den Noort JC, Scholtes VA, Harlaar J (2009) Evaluation of clinical spasticity assessment in cerebral palsy using inertial sensors. *Gait & posture* **30**: 138–143.

Novak I, Morgan C, Adde L et al. (2017) Early, Accurate Diagnosis and Early Intervention in Cerebral Palsy. *JAMA Pediatrics* **171**: 897–907.

Novak I, Morgan C, Fahey M et al. (2020) State of the Evidence Traffic Lights 2019: Systematic Review of Interventions for Preventing and Treating Children with Cerebral Palsy. *Curr Neurol Neurosci Rep* **20**: 1–21.

Ostensjø S, Carlberg EB, Vøllestad NK (2004) Motor impairments in young children with cerebral palsy: Relationship to gross motor function and everyday activities. *Dev Med Child Neurol* **46**: 580–589.

Palisano RJ, Rosenbaum P, Bartlett D, Livingston MH (2008) Content validity of the expanded and revised Gross Motor Function Classification System. *Developmental Medicine and Child Neurology* **50**: 744–750.

Pandyan AD, Johnson GR, Price CI, Curless RH, Barnes MP, Rodgers H (1999) A review of the properties and limitations of the Ashworth and modified Ashworth Scales as measures of spasticity. *Clin Rehabil* **13**: 373–383.

Pandyan AD, Price CI, Rodgers H, Barnes MP, Johnson GR (2001) Biomechanical examination of a commonly used measure of spasticity/. *Clin Biomech* **16**: 859–865.

Pandyan AD, Van Wijck FM, Stark S, Vuadens P, Johnson GR, Barnes MP (2006) The construct validity of a spasticity measurement device for clinical practice: an alternative to the Ashworth scales. *Disabil Rehabil* **28**: 579–585.

Pavone L, Burton J, Gaebler-Spira D (2013) Dystonia in Childhood. *Journal of Child Neurology* **28**: 340–350.

Platz T, Eickhof C, Nuyens G, Vuadens P (2005) Clinical scales for the assessment of spasticity, associated phenomena, and function: a systematic review of the literature. *Disabil and Rehabil* **27**: 7–18.

Rice J and Waugh MC (2009) Pilot study on trihexyphenidyl in the treatment of dystonia in children with cerebral palsy. *J Child Neurol* **24**: 176–182.

Ross SA and Engsberg JR (2007) Relationships Between Spasticity, Strength, Gait, and the GMFM-66 in Persons With Spastic Diplegia Cerebral Palsy. *Arch Phys Med Rehabil* **88**: 1114–1120.

Sanger TD, Delgado MR, Gaebler-Spira D, Hallett M, Mink JW, Task Force on Childhood Motor Disorders (2003) Classification and definition of disorders causing hypertonia in childhood. *Pediatrics* **111**: e89–e97.

Sanger TD, Chen D, Delgado MR, Gaebler-Spira D, Hallett M, Mink JW; Taskforce on Childhood Motor Disorders (2006) Definition and classification of negative motor signs in childhood. *Pediatrics* **118**: 2159–2167.

Schless SH, Desloovere K, Aertbeliën E, Molenaers G, Huenaerts C, Bar-On L (2015) The intra- and inter-rater reliability of an instrumented spasticity assessment in children with cerebral palsy. *PLoS ONE* **10**: e0131011

Schwartz MH, Rozumalski A, Trost JP (2008) The effect of walking speed on the gait of typically developing children. *J Biomech* **41**: 1639–1650.

Sinkjaer T, Toft E, Larsen K, Andreassen S, Hansen HJ (1993) Non-reflex and reflex mediated ankle joint stiffness in multiple sclerosis patients with spasticity. *Muscle nerve* **16**: 69–76.

Sloot LH, Bar-On L, van der Krogt MM et al. (2017) Motorized versus manual instrumented spasticity assessment in children with cerebral palsy. *Dev Med Child Neurol* **59**: 145–151.

Smith LR, Chambers HG, Subramaniam S, Lieber RL (2012) Transcriptional abnormalities of hamstring muscle contractures in children with cerebral palsy. *PLoS ONE* **7**: e40686.

Smith LR, Chambers HG, Lieber RL (2013) Reduced satellite cell population may lead to contractures in children with cerebral palsy. *Dev Med Child Neurol* **55**: 264–270.

Stansfield BW, Hillman SJ, Hazlewood ME et al. (2001) Sagittal joint kinematics, moments, and powers are predominantly characterized by speed of progression, not age, in normal children. *J Pediatr Orthop* **21**: 403–411.

Tardieu G, Shentoub S, DelarueE R (1954) Research on a technic for measurement of spasticity. *Revue neurologique* **91**: 143–144.

Theis N, Korff T, Mohagheghi AA (2015) Does long-term passive stretching alter muscle-tendon unit mechanics in children with spastic cerebral palsy? *Clin Biomech* **30**: 1071–1076.

Theis N, Mohagheghi AA, Korff T (2016) Mechanical and material properties of the plantarflexor muscles and Achilles tendon in children with spastic cerebral palsy and typically developing children. *J Biomech* **49**: 3004–3008.

Tuzson AE, Granata KP, Abel MF (2003) Spastic velocity threshold constrains functional performance in cerebral palsy. *Arch Phys Med Rehabil* **84**: 1363–1368.

Vanmechelen I, Bekteshi S, Bossier K, Feys H, Deklerck J, Monbaliu E (2019) Presence and severity of dystonia and choreoathetosis overflow movements in participants with dyskinetic cerebral palsy and their relation with functional classification scales. *Disabil Rehabil* **42**: 1548–1555.

Vanmechelen I, Dan B, Feys H, Monbaliu E (2020) Test–retest reliability of the Dyskinesia Impairment Scale: measuring dystonia and choreoathetosis in dyskinetic cerebral palsy. *Dev Med Child Neurol* **62**: 489–493.

Vidailhet M, Yelnik J, Lagrange C et al.; French SPIDY-2 Study Group (2009) Bilateral pallidal deep brain stimulation for the treatment of patients with dystonia-choreoathetosis cerebral palsy: a prospective pilot study. *Lancet Neurol* **8**: 709–717.

de Vlugt E, de Groot JH, Schenkeveld KE, Arendzen JH, van der Helm FC, Meskers CG (2010) The relation between neuromechanical parameters and Ashworth score in stroke patients. *J Neuroeng Rehabil* **7**: 5–7.

de Vlugt E, de Groot JH, Wisman WH, Meskers CG (2012) Clonus is explained from increased reflex gain and enlarged tissue viscoelasticity. *J Biomech* **45**: 148–155.

Voerman GE, Gregoric M, Hermens HJ (2005) Neurophysiological methods for the assessment of spasticity: the Hoffmann reflex, the tendon reflex, and the stretch reflex. *Disabil Rehabil* **27**: 33–68.

WHO (2020) International Classification of Functioning, Disability and Health (ICF) *WHO*. World Health Organization.

Willaert J, Desloovere K, Van Campenhout A, Ting LH, De Groote F (2020) Movement history influences pendulum kinematics in children with spastic cerebral palsy. *Frontiers in bioengineering and biotechnology* **8**: 920.

Willerslev-Olsen M, Lorentzen J, Sinkjaer T, Nielsen JB (2013) Passive muscle properties are altered in children with cerebral palsy before the age of 3 years and are difficult to distinguish clinically from spasticity. *Dev Med Child Neurol* **55**: 617–623.

Willerslev-Olsen M, Andersen JB, Sinkjaer T, Nielsen JB (2014) Sensory feedback to ankle plantar flexors is not exaggerated during gait in spastic hemiplegic children with cerebral palsy. *J Neurophysiol* **111**: 746–754.

Wood DE, Burridge JH, van Wijck FM et al. (2005) Biomechanical approaches applies to the lower and upper limb for the measurement of spasticity: A systematic review of the literature. *Disabil Rehabil* **27**: 19–32.

Wu YN, Ren Y, Goldsmith A, Gaebler D, Liu SQ, Zhang LQ (2010) Characterization of spasticity in cerebral palsy: dependence of catch angle on velocity. *Dev Med Child Neurol* **52**: 563–569.

Yamaguchi T, Hvass Petersen T, Kirk H et al. (2018) Spasticity in adults with cerebral palsy and multiple sclerosis measured by objective clinically applicable technique. *Clin Neurophysiol* **129**: 2010–2021.

Zhou JY, Lowe E, Cahill-Rowlwy K, Mahtani GBB, Young JL, Rose J (2019) Influence of impaired selective motor control on gait in children with cerebral palsy. *Journal of Children's Orthopaedics* **13**: 73–81.

Spasticity and Dystonia
Consequences, Management, and Future Perspectives

Kristina Tedroff and Marjolein van der Krogt

KEY POINTS

- Historically, much emphasis on the treatment of children with cerebral palsy (CP) has been on spasticity reduction, but the effects of current treatments on daily life functioning are lacking or highly variable.
- Botulinum neurotoxin A (BoNT-A) and selective dorsal rhizotomy (SDR) should be applied in well-selected patients only.
- Scientific evidence on the treatment of dystonia in ambulatory patients with CP is almost completely lacking.
- Better outcome assessment of current treatment options as well as a search for novel treatment modalities is crucial.

OPPORTUNITIES

- Single-subject, multiple baseline designs to study the effects of spasticity and dystonia treatment can yield high-level evidence and are more feasible in clinical practice than randomized controlled trial (RCT) designs.
- Novel techniques in gait analysis and gait training allow for better assessment of the dynamic effects of spasticity in more challenging conditions and open up new opportunities for advanced training.
- Better (ambulant) measurement of dystonia will allow for improved monitoring of treatment effects and assessment of the potential confounding effect of dystonia on treatment outcomes in patients with mixed CP types.

From a motor control perspective, cerebral palsy (CP) is best described as a set of different motor disorders with motor dysfunction that varies in range and type. For simplicity, these symptoms have been categorized as excess symptoms, which are added onto normal motor behavior, and deficit symptoms, in which the typical motor repertoire fails to develop (Forssberg 2003). Among the excess symptoms, spasticity and dystonia have traditionally been considered to be the most common and debilitating. Consequently, much focus has been placed on reducing or eliminating these symptoms in ambulatory children with CP.

The most common subtypes of CP are spastic CP, affecting 80% to 90%, and dyskinetic CP, reported in 5% to 11% when large population-based samples have been classified, such as in the Nordic countries ('Yearly report CPUP' 2019). Dyskinetic CP includes different forms of dyskinesia: dystonia, athetosis, and chorea. Furthermore, as in children with primarily spastic CP, dystonia can occur as a secondary symptom, and this co-occurrence of dyskinesia in spastic CP has recently received increased attention. In a study from Australia, 151 children, of which 85% were classified as spastic type, were evaluated for dystonia through a comprehensive protocol (Rice et al. 2017). The study found that ~80% and ~60% of children with primarily spastic type CP had dystonia of the lower and upper limbs respectively (Rice et al. 2017).

The primary treatment options to reduce the effects of spasticity are the use of botulinum neurotoxin A (BoNT-A) (often combined with serial casting and intensive therapy), selective dorsal rhizotomy (SDR), and oral or intrathecal baclofen (ITB) treatment. Common treatment options for dystonia in CP include focal BoNT-A and oral medication. Deep brain stimulation (DBS) is also used more regularly to treat dystonia of hereditary type, but its use in CP is limited.

This chapter briefly summarizes what is known about the long-term effects of spasticity and dystonia and the evidence base for some of the more often used treatment options for spasticity and dystonia, with a main focus on ambulatory children with CP. We aim to identify knowledge gaps in this current evidence and describe our proposed direction of research to fill these gaps. Furthermore, we highlight several novel, emerging treatment options and their potential to supplement or replace conventional treatment. Finally, several preferred research goals for the coming 5 years are listed.

SPASTICITY: CONSEQUENCES AND CURRENT MANAGEMENT

Spasticity in CP mainly hampers voluntary movements, but it has been argued (without scientific support) that spasticity may sometimes be helpful for the weak child when, for example, spasticity of the lower extremities may assist weight-bearing or support. Severe spasticity can be both painful and can lead to increased energy consumption, which is thought to be one of the factors contributing to the growth disturbances often seen in CP (Hemingway et al. 2001). Some assumptions are commonly made concerning the relationship between spasticity and aspects of functioning in CP. These are: spasticity is believed to negatively correlate with functioning, and spasticity is frequently referred to as a major cause of development of contractures. In this section, we will discuss these assumptions.

When evaluating the consequences of spasticity, it is useful to remember that spasticity exists in a range of different conditions such as multiple sclerosis, hereditary spastic paraparesis, after stroke, and after traumatic brain injury or spinal cord injury occurring after 2 years of age. Depending on the etiology, many aspects of spasticity vary, and consequently, when we address spasticity in CP we can only use the knowledge obtained from individuals with CP.

Fully understanding the natural development of spasticity is crucial when evaluating long-term effects of development as well as possible complications. Over the last years, studies that have used a large population-based registry, the Swedish surveillance program for CP ('Yearly report CPUP'), comprising of greater than 95% of all children with CP in Sweden, have been able to display information pertinent to long-term or natural development of spasticity in children with CP (Franzen et al. 2017; Linden et al. 2019). In a longitudinal cohort study, 4162 children with CP, born between 1990 and 2015, were evaluated through repeated standardized follow-up examinations. In total, ~58 000 measurements of spasticity

(Ashworth scale) of the gastrocsoleus were reported (Linden et al. 2019). The main findings of the study were that the degree of spasticity increased in most children during their first 5 years of life, followed by a decrease during the remaining follow-up periods up to 15 years of age (Fig. 5.1). When children who had had SDR (*n*=65), ITB (*n*=67), or Achilles tendon lengthening (*n*=430) were excluded from the analysis, findings were somewhat attenuated, but the same trends of spasticity development were observed (Linden et al. 2019).

Findings supporting this natural decrease in spasticity were reported in another study from the same registry evaluating the use of BoNT-A at different ages (Franzen et al. 2017). While the proportion of those that had BoNT-A treatment during the study period 2010 to 2015 remained stable, significantly fewer children had BoNT-A treatment at later ages. The proportion treated with BoNT-A varied with age and peaked at 4 to 6 years. The odds ratio of having had BoNT-A treatment were 2.02 for the 4 to 6 year olds (treatment within the preceding 6–12mo) and 0.81 for the 13 to 15 year olds (treatment within the preceding 12–24mo). This indicates that most children receive BoNT-A treatment when they are likely to have the highest degree of spasticity (Franzen et al. 2017).

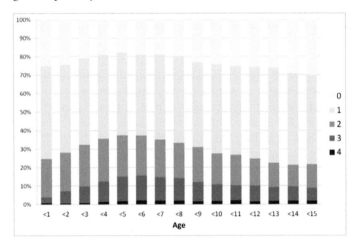

Figure 5.1 Degree of spasticity in the gastrocnemius-soleus according to Modified Ashworth Scale related to age in the total sample. Number of measurements presented as a percentage of the total number of measurements in each age group. Adapted from Linden et al. 2019 with permission from Taylor & Francis on behalf of the Nordic Orthopedic Federation.

Consequences of Spasticity

Studies that evaluated the etiology of pain in CP are scarce, but it has been suggested that increased muscle tone, i.e. spasticity and dystonia, is a possible cause of pain (Barwood et al. 2000). As a consequence, spasticity reducing interventions have been reported to reduce pain caused by muscle spasm (Multani et al. 2019; Tedroff et al. 2019a). In the clinical setting, the treatment of pain in children with CP with repeated cycles of BoNT-A is common, more so in non-ambulant patients (Tedroff et al. 2018). Furthermore, increased energy expenditure secondary to spasticity has been shown in a few studies (Hemingway et al. 2001; Balaban et al. 2012; Saxena et al. 2016).

One of the crucial questions, however, is whether spasticity negatively affects (daily life) function in CP. This classic assumption has important meaning for the indication and development of many interventions. Today, some evidence supports the notion that reduced function is not a consequence of spasticity, and that reducing spasticity will not correspond in a predictive, clinically meaningful, and persistent increase in function (Multani et al. 2019; Tedroff et al. 2019b). Ross and Engsberg conducted a study where spasticity, strength, and functional outcome, as assessed by Gross Motor Function Measure (GMFM-66) and a range of gait analysis parameters, were tested in 97 children with CP and Gross Motor Function Classification System (GMFCS) levels I to III (2007). They found that spasticity only accounted for a maximum of 8% of the variance in gait and gross motor function, whereas moderate to high correlations were found between strength and these functions, accounting for up to 69% of the variance.

In a seminal paper, Novak and co-authors evaluated 64 discrete interventions in CP in a systematic review (Novak et al. 2013). Interventions were evaluated using the Oxford Levels of Evidence; GRADE (Grading of Recommendations, Assessment, Development, and Evaluations); Evidence Alert Traffic Light; and the International Classification of Function, Disability, and Health systems. Pertinent to spasticity, the authors found that BoNT-A, SDR, and diazepam were effective in reducing spasticity in themselves, all having a recommendation of 'do it' with a high level of evidence. However, evidence for improvements in motor activities, or function, and self-care, is less strong, and high-quality studies are lacking. Hence, the overall level of evidence was weak and situated between 'effect unknown' and 'probably do it' (Novak et al. 2013). Hence, the exact relevance of spasticity during functional tasks still remains unclear, including spasticity in relation to other impairments such as limited selective motor control or weakness.

Another topic of controversy is whether spasticity, in turn, leads to muscle contractures. When relaxed muscles fail to reach 'normal length' or a length appropriate for the bone, we talk about contractures. Consequently, contractures will reduce joint range of motion for the joint(s), which they span. As of today, knowledge of the specific mechanisms underlying the development of contractures and the difficulty in preventing them is at its best incomplete (Multani et al. 2019). There are, however, many assumptions in clinical practice as well as the literature that links spasticity to contractures, often claiming that spasticity causes it. It is known that two of the interventions that most effectively reduce or even remove spasticity in the child with CP, BoNT-A, and SDR, do not completely prevent contractures from forming (Multani et al. 2019; Tedroff et al. 2019b).

In an attempt to evaluate the effect on contracture formation and the need for orthopedic surgery following the most potent intervention aimed at reducing spasticity, SDR, a figure was constructed to show the prevalence of orthopedic surgery in the years after SDR (Fig. 5.2). This figure illustrates the proportion of individuals included in an SDR follow-up study that reported the need for orthopedic surgery after SDR and the time in years after the neurosurgical intervention. Although not all studies reported orthopedic surgery consistently and did not always differentiate soft tissue surgery from bony surgery, many did state that soft tissue surgery was prevalent. It is obvious from this figure that there is a near-linear relationship between time after SDR and the percentage of individuals that have had orthopedic surgery. These findings illustrate that contractures still often occur after SDR, supporting the idea that factors other than spasticity can lead to contractures. Hence, the exact relationship between spasticity and the forming of contractures is not yet fully understood.

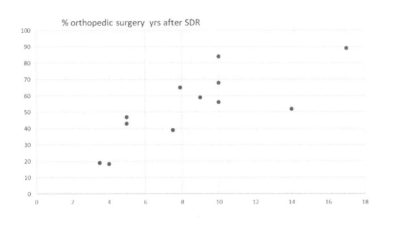

| 17y Tedroff 2015 |
| 14y Ailon 2015 |
| 10y Bolster 2013 (55%) |
| 10y Tedroff 2011 (84%) |
| 10y Romei 2018 (42%) |
| 9y McFall 2015 |
| 7,9y Carroll 1998 |
| 7,5y O'Brien 2005 |
| 5y Arens 1989 (47%) |
| 5y Nordmark 2008 (42%) |
| 4y Mittal 2002 |
| 3,5y Chicoine 1997 |

Figure 5.2 Prevalence of orthopedic surgery in years after selective dorsal rhizotomy (SDR) x-axis = years post SDR. y-axis = % of participants having had orthopedic surgeries after their SDR. Every marker = 1 study. For 5 and 10 years after surgery the percentage of the specific study is stated in the textbox.

Treatment of Spasticity

When aiming to reduce or eliminate spasticity in CP, the fundamental question is: are current interventions effective, and if so, in what aspect (Novak et al. 2013)? Second, it is useful to consider if that aspect is important for the intended child. In CP, clinical trial results that clearly support a specific therapy are scarce. Generally speaking, therapy can be divided into rehabilitation management, medical management with oral and local therapy, and surgical interventions (either neurosurgical or orthopedic). In this section, we will specifically focus on two of the more common, muscle tone reducing, and to some extent, controversial interventions, BoNT-A and SDR.

BoNT-A

BoNT-A is the most common treatment to reduce spasticity in children with CP, typically aiming to improve ambulatory function in those in GMFCS levels I to III. Since the first publication in 1993, there was a rapid transformation from basic research to clinical practice, and usage almost exploded. Although, early on, this wide-spread use was argued to be too common due to the lack of treatment standardization, and limited follow-up time for most clinical studies at the time (Forssberg and Tedroff 1997; Gough et al. 2005; Reddihough et al. 2002). As stated above, Novak et al. in 2013 categorized the use of BoNT-A as 'do it', with good evidence for improvements in spasticity, although effects on daily-life functioning were less clear. Today, several Cochrane library systematic reviews with meta-analyses have been published, most recently an update by Blumetti et al. (2019). This Cochrane review, including 31 randomized controlled trials and ~1500 children, concludes that

'The quality of the evidence was low or very low for most of the outcomes analyzed. We found limited evidence that BoNT-A is more effective than placebo or a non-placebo control at improving gait, joint range of motion, satisfaction, and lower limb spasticity in children with CP, whereas the results for function were contradictory'.

Importantly, most of the published studies have short follow-up periods (3–6mo) and have evaluated one treatment cycle only (Tedroff 2009; Blumetti et al. 2019; Multani et al. 2019), an insufficient approach when evaluating long-term effect or harm. In addition, a recent comprehensive narrative review by Multani et al. (2019) emphasized that some of the differences in outcomes in clinical trials may relate to the use of adjunctive interventions such as serial casting, orthoses, night splints, and intensive therapy. Supporting this are the findings of a recent Dutch study reporting that BoNT-A before a comprehensive rehabilitation program has no added value to goal attainment or gait kinematics (Schasfoort et al. 2018).

There are other indications for BoNT-A, such as potentially delaying orthopedic surgery (Desloovere et al. 2007), improved orthotics use, or pain reduction, which can be relevant in some patient cases. Pain is frequently reported in all children with CP, across GMFCS levels and subtypes (Tervo et al. 2006). In a real-world study, which included all children with CP (*n*=159) in the Greater Stockholm area that received BoNT-A during a 16 month period, pain reduction was the second most common treatment, reported in 31% of all cases many being ambulatory (Tedroff et al. 2018). However, when BoNT-A is also used for pain reduction, the results are conflicting and overall level of evidence is low (Ostojic et al. 2019).

In a recent comprehensive narrative review on BoNT-A use in CP the authors concluded that clinical protocols for BoNT-A use in children with CP needs to be revised and include longitudinal monitoring of the specific effects on muscle morphology (Multani et al. 2019). Further, they reported that studies, including small numbers of healthy volunteers or larger studies in experimental animals, had observed muscle atrophy detectable for at least 12 months after BoNT-A injections. Evidence from animal studies suggests that BoNT-A injections might cause loss of contractile elements and increased fibrosis, possibly increasing contracture development (Minamoto et al. 2015; Ward et al. 2018). No longitudinal study exists that has specifically evaluated the long-term development of these muscular changes, and currently, we do not know if they are reversible (Multani et al. 2019), nor if they occur in humans. All in all, these findings justify a careful use of BoNT-A in children with CP, considering both the available evidence for beneficial treatment effects as well as potential risks.

SDR

SDR has been used fairy regularly for children with spastic CP for four decades. Despite being used in all GMFCS levels, most centers recommend the procedure for children that have some level of ambulatory function (GMFCS levels I–III). The subject of SDR is quite polarized between those that recommend and those that avoid the procedure. Some centers conduct large numbers of procedures annually, while others offer the procedure to a small number of patients fulfilling strict inclusion criteria. While some centers have discontinued this intervention altogether.

In SDR, a careful selection of sensory afferent fibers are cut when entering the spinal cord, typically reducing, or even eliminating, lower limb spasticity with the aim of improving function and activities. During the 21st century, much emphasis has been put on establishing what type of children will benefit the most from the procedure and to establish the type of assessment tools that can most appropriately identify treatment effects. In this section, we report on the level of evidence for the effect of SDR from the short-term (up to 2y), medium-term (5y or more), and long-term (10y or more) perspective, based on some key systematic review papers.

In 2002, Mc Laughlin and co-authors published a review and meta-analysis of three studies where SDR and physiotherapy were compared to physiotherapy only. Follow-up for these studies were 9, 12, and 24 months. Overall results showed that physiotherapy plus SDR was weakly superior to physiotherapy only with a mean change score in GMFM-66 of 2.6 at 12 months after SDR (McLaughlin et al. 2002).

When the long-term effects 5 or more years after SDR were evaluated in a systematic review, the reviewers were only able to include one study with low level of evidence (Grunt et al. 2011). The included study evaluated function and activity after SDR plus physiotherapy, and after physiotherapy only, and found equal outcomes in the two groups.

A systematic review that included individuals with CP only and 10 or more years of follow-up was published in 2019 (Tedroff et al. 2019a). Of all 16 studies that were identified and included, 14 were case series and two compared the individuals with CP to a retrospectively assigned comparison group, one of the case series compared the GMFM-66 measures to centiles in GMFM motor curves. According to the Oxford Centre for Evidence-based Medicine, the level of evidence of included studies was low, two at level 3 and 14 at level 4. The overall risk of bias was medium-to-high in all cases. All of the included sample sizes were small (n=11–95), being less than 50 in 13 of the 16 studies. There were considerable differences in study design, clinical variability between the research populations, loss to follow-up, and heterogeneity across trials, aspects that prevented a meta-analysis approach. The authors concluded that

'at ≥10 years of follow-up available studies generate low-level evidence with considerable bias. No functional improvement of SDR over routine therapy is documented. Furthermore, long-term effects of SDR with respect to spasticity reduction is unclear, with many studies reporting a high amount of add-on spasticity treatment'.

Only 7 out of 16 studies appraised the effect on spasticity in particular, and all of these reported sustained long-term reduction or even normal muscle tone (Tedroff et al. 2019b). However, five studies, including two of those that documented long-term reduction in spasticity noted a need for additional spasticity treatment such as BoNT-A (45%–59%), ITB, or oral treatment. Altogether, 28% to 94% of all the included patients underwent orthopedic surgery subsequent to SDR, often soft tissue surgery to correct contractures. The most common functional outcome was GMFM, reported in six studies that all reported an early increase, however only two of those made comparisons to the expected changes in GMFM as earlier illustrated in the GMFM motor curves (Hanna et al. 2008).

Of particular interest was a study by Munger and coworkers (2017) that made retrospective comparisons (indicated by a propensity model to be highly accurate) of 24 individuals that had SDR to a comparison group of 11 individuals whose clinical presentation was appropriate for SDR, but who, for a variety of reasons, did not undergo surgery (Munger et al. 2017). This study reported that when gait was evaluated through gait analysis and the gait deviation index (GDI), individuals that did not undergo SDR had a larger improvement in gait after 10 years, compared to the group that had SDR, but had significantly more interventions (Munger et al. 2017). The authors suggested that differing treatment courses provide similar outcomes into early adulthood (Munger et al. 2017).

From the above, it is clear that further long-term follow-up with scientifically sound protocols or large registry data is needed to better quantify the positive and adverse effects of SDR and identify in which patients the procedure works best.

DYSTONIA: CONSEQUENCES AND CURRENT MANAGEMENT

Dyskinetic CP is only reported in 5% to 11% of all individuals with CP. The rareness of the condition is likely a contributing factor to the present situation where neither the long-term effects secondary to dystonia or choreoathetosis or effective treatments are known. It is easy to grasp when the following calculation is made. In a population that includes 100 000 children 0 to 18 years of age, an estimate of 250 will have CP. Out of those, ~20 will have dyskinetic CP, and the majority, 60% to 65%, will be in GMFCS levels IV or V. Thus only eight children of all ages will be ambulatory dyskinetic CP (Himmelmann et al. 2009; Surveillance of Cerebral Palsy in Europe 2000). However, as stated above, dystonia may also be highly frequent as a secondary condition in spastic CP (Rice et al. 2017), which highlights the relevance to better understand this condition.

Individuals with CP and dyskinetic symptoms such as chorea, athetosis, or dystonia, have pathological movements that are often seen when initiating a movement. Dystonia is characterized by abnormal stereotyped shifts in muscle tone and muscle co-contraction. It is often induced by movement or external stimuli. Voluntary movements may be distorted, or movements may be involuntary. Affected muscles or limbs may 'freeze' in abnormal positions or postures, often characterized by rotation, extension, or flexion. Children with hyperkinetic or choreoathetotic CP are severely hampered in motor activity by extensive involuntary movements and overflow of muscle activity to muscle groups other than those intended (Graham et al. 2016).

Consequences of Dystonia

In CP, many comorbid features often co-occurring with dystonia are known, such as dysphagia, dysarthria, pain, and sleep problems (Himmelmann et al. 2009; Tedroff et al. 2019a). From a study evaluating the effect of SDR in non-ambulatory patients with severe bilateral spasticity, we have learned that if the reduction of spasticity after SDR unveils dystonia, parents tend to be much less pleased with the surgery (van de Pol et al. 2018). However, consequences secondary to dystonia specific to gait or ambulation have hardly been described only very minimally (Davids et al. 1999; Abel et al. 2003). No observational prospective nor retrospective study exists that describes the long-term effects of dystonia in CP.

Treatment of Dyskinetic CP

Few studies have specifically focused on the treatment of dystonia in dyskinetic CP, and to the best of our knowledge, no study has targeted ambulatory children with dyskinetic CP. Most studies reporting on interventions in dystonia in CP included a wide span of differing conditions, not only CP, that display dystonia, and some conditions will even be progressive. This is less appropriate since treatment effects are closely related to the specific etiology of the dystonia (Danielsson et al. 2019). Additionally, age spans are often wide, sometimes including young children, school-aged children, adolescents, and adults. All in all, the evidence is lacking for effective treatment of the dyskinetic features in CP.

During a search of the Cochrane library, only one review aimed at evaluating the effect of treatment in dyskinetic CP was identified. This review specifically evaluated the effect of oral trihexyphenidyl in dyskinetic CP dystonia. Furthermore, only one study was identified for the review; a randomized controlled trial (RCT) including 16 participants, with only two ambulatory patients in GMFCS level II, and 14 in GMFCS levels IV or V, the level of evidence was low, and a high risk of side effects was reported (Harvey et al. 2018).

Another recent systematic (non-Cochrane) review that specifically evaluated the effect of oral or neurosurgical interventions in dyskinetic CP included 28 studies that were classified according to their study design but not evaluated for level of bias (Fehlings et al. 2018). Although most of the included studies reported dyskinesia secondary to many differing etiologies, studies were excluded if less than 50% of the reported individuals had CP and if these individuals were not clearly identifiable and if results were presented for this subsample. The review concluded that 'Current evidence does not support the effectiveness of oral medications or BoNT-A in reducing dystonia and the use of these interventions is based on clinical expert opinion. There is generally inadequate evidence to evaluate the pharmacological and neurosurgical interventions' impact on motor function, pain relief, or ease of caregiving, as well as evidence guiding the sequencing or combining of therapies', but 'ITB and DBS are possibly effective in reducing dystonia'

(Fehlings et al. 2018). Recently, Bonouvrié et al. (2019) published an RCT in 36 patients with severe dyskinetic CP (GMFCS levels IV–V), showing that ITB is superior to placebo in achieving treatment goals.

Although there are very few studies that evaluate the effect of different interventions for dyskinetic CP, in clinical practice some treatments, discussed below, are often used and would deserve better scientific evaluation. BoNT-A has been used for focal primary or hereditary dystonia for more than 40 years. It effectively reduces muscle tone, reduces pain, and increases patient-reported quality of life (Castelao et al. 2017). In dyskinetic CP, the evidence is lacking, but BoNT-A is often used if dystonia is focal or painful. Furthermore, a range of different oral drugs can be evaluated, but the treatment effect is often disappointing and side effects substantial. Baclofen and trihexyphenidyl are some of the more commonly used oral drugs, and in some patients, they provide limited and transient improvement (Roubertie et al. 2012; Fehlings et al. 2018). The use of orthotics can be effective in some instances with dystonia. However, for some individuals, the pressure from the orthotic device can result in an unwanted increase in dystonia, and for others, the usage can be painful due to the often-strong forces associated with dystonia.

DBS

During the 21st century, much hope has been put into the possibility of reducing motor symptoms in dyskinetic CP through the use of neurosurgically administered DBS. DBS is a well-established, although invasive, intervention for dystonia, as well as for other movement disorders, such as essential tremor and Parkinson disorder (Danielsson et al. 2019). If dystonia is isolated and generalized, DBS will have good and occasionally even excellent results, with motor improvement ranging from 50% to 75% when assessed by a variety of methods (Vidailhet et al. 2007). On the other hand, the outcome of DBS in individuals with dystonia in combination with other neurological symptoms or an abnormal brain magnetic resonance imaging scan such as in dyskinetic CP is less predictable, often resulting in little or no improvement (Elkaim et al. 2019).

Specifically, for dyskinetic CP, DBS was first used in 2000 (Koy et al. 2013). A couple of dozen studies have been published, but many are case reports and 11 original publications each report on a single patient. The same patients are also reported on in different publications. All in all, the exact number of individuals that have been reported on is hard to establish but likely does not exceed 140 unique patients with dyskinetic CP up until 2019 (Koy et al. 2013; Elia et al. 2018; Fehlings et al. 2018). Very few of these individuals are ambulatory. Three systematic reviews exist, but only one of those include patients with dyskinetic CP only (Koy et al. 2013; Elia et al. 2018; Fehlings et al. 2018). The level of evidence for the reported effect is very low and the risk of bias in all studies is high.

In 2019, Tustin and co-authors reported on a series of pediatric patients with dystonia of varied etiology from the same London facility (Tustin et al. 2019). This study included spaghetti-plots grouped by etiology reporting on GMFM-88 and the Burke–Fahn–Marsden Dystonia Rating Scale-Movement scale, that is somewhat similar to the single-subject study design, is illustrating the effect. In total 131 children had received DBS, but the study excluded all those that had technical issues or had their DBS removed, thus leaving 60 children that were followed for 2 years. Twenty of these children had acquired dystonia, and 19 were identified as having CP (16 out of 19 in GMFCS levels IV–V). For this specific group, median GMFM-88 and Burke–Fahn–Marsden Dystonia Rating Scale-movement change scores were near zero at the 2 year follow-up (Tustin et al. 2019). The authors stated that 'expectations for significant gross motor function change following DBS should be tempered when goal setting for children with CP' (Tustin et al. 2019). Hence, currently, the overall evidence base does not support the use of DBS in dyskinetic CP.

FUTURE DIRECTIONS (1): IMPROVE OUTCOME ASSESSMENT OF CURRENT TREATMENT OPTIONS

From the above, it is clear that better and higher level of evidence for current spasticity and dystonia management is warranted. As of yet, no studies have been able to show clear added value of BoNT-A on activity or participation measures, and the effects of SDR have been mixed at best. In case no clear treatment effects can be demonstrated, these treatments should be reevaluated, or only performed for specific subgroups where benefits are clearer. To better assess treatment outcomes, RCT's can yield the highest level of evidence, but are difficult to execute in CP due to the heterogeneity in patient characteristics as well as in treatment options and may also raise ethical concerns.

An alternative test design which may be much more feasible in CP but has not yet been used much, is the repeated baseline single-subject research design. In this approach, the participant serves as their own control, and differences before and after treatment are compared to natural progression over a similar time period before the treatment is started. A repeated baseline assessment can be embedded as part of clinical practice by postponing treatment or taking advantage of existing waiting lists. Several types of single-subject research designs can be carried out, including simple baseline designs (A–B) or replicated baseline designs (ABA, with a follow-up period after treatment, or ABC, in which C is a second treatment option), or cross-over designs. When performed with blinded measurements and random allocation of treatments, such designs are considered to yield the highest level of evidence (Romeiser Logan et al. 2008), requiring fewer participants than typical RCT designs. An example of a successful implementation of repeated-baseline design is the study by Van Vulpen et al. (2017; 2018), showing that functional power training yields better improvements in walking capacity, personalized treatment goals, and parent-reported mobility performance compared with a similar period of usual care in young children with CP. We propose implementing this type of design to better assess the short-term outcomes of SDR, BoNT-A, and baclofen treatment in CP.

In cases where repeated baselines are not possible, or to assess long-term outcomes, standardized registering of treatment effects in regular clinical care should be improved as well. Such registration can be done in individual centers using standardized treatment protocols with fixed pre- and post-measurements, but much stronger outcome assessment will be possible when data is combined in national or international treatment registries (such as in the annual 'Yearly report from CPUP'). This allows for data pooling, outcome assessment over larger groups of patients, comparison of outcomes between centers and different treatment modalities, as well as to identify predicting factors for good or poor treatment outcomes. Furthermore, by registering patient development over time, better cohorts for typical development should be generated, which can serve as a reference to compare individual patient's treatment effects.

In any type of research design or standardized outcome assessment, it is of utmost importance to include outcome measures of all ICF-CY (International Classification of Functioning, Disability, and Health - Child and Youth) domains. Measures at structure and function level are essential to help us understand the working mechanisms of treatments. For instance, in the case of BoNT-A treatment, outcome assessment should include evaluation of the (long-term) changes in muscle morphology, to better assess the potentially detrimental effect of BoNT-A on muscle health. Simple measures of functional capacity, such as timed up and go test or 1-minute walk test, should be easy to implement and could serve as reliable and relevant outcomes to obtain for large groups of participants. At the other end of the ICF-CY spectrum, patient-reported outcomes, and health-related quality of life measures are essential to capture the actual benefits of treatment for patients and their parents in daily life. For this purpose, we recommend including measures such as Goal Attainment Scaling (Turner-Stokes 2009) and Gait Outcomes Assessment List (Thomason et al. 2018) in any treatment evaluation.

5-YEAR PRIORITY #1:

- Better evaluation of SDR and BoNT-A treatment outcomes using repeated-baseline designs and/or data harmonization and pooling, including outcome measures at all domains of the ICF-CY.

Given the heterogeneity of the CP population, an individual's treatment success is highly dependent on the proper selection of the right treatment for the right patient. This treatment selection is a complicated process, typically starting with patient need and incorporating data from consultation, physical examination, and gait analysis. This process is performed differently in different centers, leading to differences in diagnosing the underlying problems and in treatment selections. Hence, better standardization and clarification of this clinical reasoning process is required.

One aspect that may improve the clinical reasoning process would be a better unraveling of the underlying impairments during gait. While gait analysis yields a wealth of information on the patient's gait abnormalities and potential underlying causes, it only reflects the patterns during a short stretch of walking under ideal circumstances. This allows for compensations masking the actual impairments, while patients also tend to select their ideal 'doctor's walk' not reflecting problems in daily life. By challenging patients more towards their limits, a much better picture of actual limitations may become visible. For instance, walking at faster walking speed exaggerates walking abnormalities, thereby better demonstrating the effects of spasticity on gait (van der Krogt et al. 2009a; van der Krogt et al. 2009b). Also walking for longer periods of time and with increased levels of fatigue may enhance, and thereby elucidate, walking abnormalities and better reflect problems in daily life (Parent et al. 2016).

Gait analysis could also be enhanced with perturbations or biofeedback, particularly when gait analysis is performed on a treadmill. It has recently been shown that treadmill perturbations can be used to evoke stretch reflexes during gait (Sloot et al. 2015), which may allow quantifying the extent of enhanced reflexes during gait in patients to better inform and evaluate spasticity treatment. Furthermore, biofeedback can be used to challenge patients in specific aspects of their gait, for instance, to increase their step length or knee extension (Booth et al. 2019), which may allow disentangling of actual impairments from compensations. Obviously, such advanced gait analysis techniques are high-end solutions only possible in specialized centers and at a high cost. These novel techniques, however, may yield insight that can be transferable to easier solutions that are also feasible in more peripheral centers.

5-YEAR PRIORITY #2:

- Develop 'smarter' assessment tools for functional effects of impairments, using more challenging tasks such as fast or fatigued walking, to better guide treatment planning and evaluation.

With respect to dyskinetic CP, treatment outcome evaluation is hampered by many factors, including the small number of patients and the large variability of symptoms. However, a key factor that limits proper outcome assessment is the lack of good, quantitative measures of dystonia. A recent review highlighted several available instrumented measures (Haberfehlner et al. 2020), but clinimetric properties are not known for any of these measures, and none of them have been accepted as routine measures in research or clinical practice. Furthermore, many measures can only be applied in lab-based environments and are time-consuming and cumbersome for the patients. Other available video-based measures, such as the Dyskinesia Impairment Scale (Monbaliu et al. 2012), also require lengthy measurements and time-consuming, offline scoring by experienced raters. As the severity of dystonia varies over time and is aggravated by external stimuli such as stress, pain, and noise (Monbaliu et al. 2017), measuring during longer periods of time in the daily situation might result in more reliable measures. Hence, novel technologies, including wearable sensors or home-based video recordings with automatic tracking, might open up new opportunities for meaningful assessment of dystonia and choreoathetosis in dyskinetic CP.

Dystonia is also an important factor to assess in patients with a primarily spastic type of CP. It was recently shown in non-ambulatory children with severe bilateral spasticity, that treatment effects were much less satisfactory when dystonia was revealed after SDR (van de Pol et al. 2018). Also, in ambulatory patients with spastic CP, the presence of dystonia as a secondary factor is commonly considered a contra-indication for several treatment options, including SDR. As dystonia may be present in up to 80% of children with spastic CP (Rice et al. 2017), this may be an important factor to affect outcomes of current spasticity treatment. However, clear guidelines or assessment methods to identify underlying dystonia in ambulatory spastic patients are lacking.

5-YEAR PRIORITY #3:

- Develop a better, standardized way of quantifying dystonia and assess whether it plays a role during walking, to better monitor treatment outcomes and quantify patients with primary and secondary symptoms of dystonia.

FUTURE DIRECTIONS (2): SEARCH FOR ALTERNATIVE TREATMENT OPTIONS

Given the limited evidence for the current spasticity management options, a search for alternative treatments is warranted. Several options have been suggested in the literature, but evidence is extremely limited, especially in CP. Here we list some of these emerging options, urging for further study on their potential in CP.

First, it has been hypothesized that eccentric exercises such as downslope walking (DSW) may lead to reduced spasticity. Several studies have investigated the effects of DSW on H-reflexes in the soleus and found reduced H-reflex activity following DSW in healthy adults (Sabatier et al. 2015; Arnold et al. 2017; Hoque et al. 2018a) as well as patients with multiple sclerosis (Hoque et al. 2018b), although not in patients post-stroke (Liang et al. 2019). Furthermore, a 6-week DSW training in persons with multiple sclerosis significantly improved walking function (Hoque et al. 2019). These findings show that DSW can induce depression of spinal reflex excitability, which shows promise for exercise interventions to reduce hyperactive reflex responses in individuals with spasticity, including those with CP.

So far, no studies have investigated the effect of eccentric exercises on spasticity or H-reflexes in CP, but some did look at other outcome measures. Hösl et al. (2018) studied the effects of backward, downhill treadmill training, which also provides eccentric stretching of the calf muscles at long muscle-tendon length. They found that backward, downhill treadmill training led to improvements in ankle dorsiflexion during gait and faster walking speeds, but no significant changes in muscle properties. Lorentzen et al. (2017) studied uphill treadmill training in adults with CP and found improvements in ankle joint stiffness, and ankle angles during gait and walking speed. Reid et al. (2010) found that eccentric strength training in the upper limb in CP greatly improved the torque-angle relationship of the elbow, possibly due to an increased number of sarcomeres in series. Altogether, these studies indicate that functional (gait) training incorporating eccentric stretching of muscles may have beneficial effects on muscle-tendon parameters, including reduction of contractures, as well as on walking capacity. Whether such training may also reduce reflexive activity in CP still has to be investigated.

An alternative type of training to reduce hyperactive reflexes is the use of operant conditioning of spinal reflexes. This approach targets plasticity to specific reflex pathways, and aims to down-regulate hyperactive reflexes through training with biofeedback on H-reflexes (Thompson et al. 2013) or stretch-reflexes (Mrachacz-Kersting et al. 2019). This approach has been very successful in reducing hyperactive reflexes and improving walking function in patients with spinal cord injury (Thompson et al. 2013). In particular, down-conditioning excessive reflexes during dynamic tasks may be most effective and beneficial (Thompson and Wolpaw 2019). However, limited evidence is available as to whether these results translate to other patient populations, including CP. Hence, further studies on neuroplasticity targeting CP are merited.

5-YEAR PRIORITY #4:

- Assess to what extent training, using eccentric exercises or operant conditioning methods, can improve (reflexive) motor control and muscle characteristics.

Finally, another therapy to reduce the effects of spasticity that has received some recent attention is the use of extracorporeal shock-wave therapy. In a recent review, Corrado et al. (2019) evaluated four studies on this topic. All four studies were of low to moderate quality but showed positive effects on Modified Ashworth scores, muscle stiffness, and joint range of motion. Hence, this warrants further study on this therapy, to assess potential benefits as well as unwanted side effects.

CONCLUSION

It is clear that better evidence for current spasticity and dystonia management should be established and novel treatment opportunities should be explored. However, it can also be questioned how relevant spasticity really is for daily-life functioning. Other factors, including impaired selective motor control, abnormal muscle function, and bone deformities may play a larger role in some patients, and hence could be a more successful target for treatment. This asks for an integrated treatment approach with a carefully tailored, patient-specific program targeting the combined set of impairments. A thorough understanding of the pathophysiology underlying spasticity, its relation to other impairments in CP, and its role during functional activities is therefore warranted.

FUTURE NEEDS:

- **Understanding the pathophysiology:** Foundational knowledge on the underlying working mechanisms of spasticity and dystonia.
- **Relative relevance of spasticity and dystonia:** Better understanding of the role of spasticity and dystonia during functional tasks, in relation to other impairments such as impaired selective motor control, contractures, weakness, and bone deformities.

REFERENCES

Abel R, Rupp R, Sutherland D (2003) Quantifying the variability of a complex motor task specifically studying the gait of dyskinetic CP children. *Gait Posture* **17**: 50–58.

Arnold E, Farmer B, Keightley M et al. (2017) Walking duration and slope steepness determine the effect of downslope walking on the soleus H-reflex pathway. *Neurosci Lett* **639**: 18–24.

Balaban B, Tok F, Tan AK, Matthews DJ (2012) Botulinum toxin a treatment in children with cerebral palsy: its effects on walking and energy expenditure. *Am J Phys Med Rehabil* **91**: 53–64.

Barwood S, Baillieu C, Boyd R et al. (2000) Analgesic effects of botulinum toxin A: a randomized, placebo-controlled clinical trial. *Dev Med Child Neurol* **42**: 116–121.

Blumetti FC, Belloti JC, Tamaoki MJ, Pinto JA (2019) Botulinum toxin type A in the treatment of lower limb spasticity in children with cerebral palsy. *Cochrane Database Syst Rev* **10**: Cd001408.

Booth AT, Buizer AI, Harlaar J, Steenbrink F, van der Krogt MM (2019) Immediate Effects of Immersive Biofeedback on Gait in Children With Cerebral Palsy. *Arch Phys Med Rehabil* **100**: 598–605.

Castelao M, Marques RE, Duarte GS et al. (2017) Botulinum toxin type A therapy for cervical dystonia. *Cochrane Database Syst Rev* **12**: CD003633.

Corrado B, Di Luise C, Servodio Iammarrone C (2019) Management of Muscle Spasticity in Children with Cerebral Palsy by Means of Extracorporeal Shockwave Therapy: A Systematic Review of the Literature. *Dev Neurorehabil* 1–7.

CPUP (2019) *Yearly report CPUP* Retrieved from http://cpup.se/wp-content/uploads/2019/10/%C3%85rsrapport-CPUP-2019-PDF.pdf

Danielsson A, Carecchio M, Cif L et al. (2019) Pallidal Deep Brain Stimulation in DYT6 Dystonia: Clinical Outcome and Predictive Factors for Motor Improvement. *J Clin Med* **8**: 2163.

Davids JR, Foti T, Dabelstein J, Blackhurst DW, Bagley A (1999) Objective assessment of dyskinesia in children with cerebral palsy. *J Pediatr Orthop* **19**: 211–214.

Desloovere K, Molenaers G, De Cat J et al. (2007) Motor function following multilevel botulinum toxin type A treatment in children with cerebral palsy. *Dev Med Child Neurol* **49**: 56–61.

Elia AE, Bagella CF, Ferré F, Zorzi G, Calandrella D, Romito LM (2018) Deep brain stimulation for dystonia due to cerebral palsy: A review. *Eur J Paediatr Neurol* **22**: 308–315.

Elkaim LM, Alotaibi NM, Sigal A et al.; North American Pediatric DBS Collaboration (2019) Deep brain stimulation for pediatric dystonia: a meta-analysis with individual participant data. *Dev Med Child Neurol* **61**: 49–56.

Fehlings D, Brown L, Harvey A et al. (2018) Pharmacological and neurosurgical interventions for managing dystonia in cerebral palsy: a systematic review. *Dev Med Child Neurol* **60**: 356–366.

Forssberg H (2003) Impaired motor programming in children with Cerebral Palsy. In R. Korinthenberg (Ed.) *Aktuelle Neurop diatrie 2002.* Nurnberg: Novartis Pharma Verlag, pp. 163–180.

Forssberg H, Tedroff KB (1997) Botulinum toxin treatment in cerebral palsy: intervention with poor evaluation? *Dev Med Child Neurol* **39**: 635–640.

Franzen M, Hagglund G, Alriksson-Schmidt A (2017) Treatment with Botulinum toxin A in a total population of children with cerebral palsy - a retrospective cohort registry study. *BMC Musculoskelet Disord* **18**: 520.

Gough M, Fairhurst C, Shortland AP (2005) Botulinum toxin and cerebral palsy: time for reflection? *Dev Med Child Neurol* **47**: 709–712.

Graham HK, Rosenbaum P, Paneth N et al. (2016) Cerebral palsy. *Nat Rev Dis Primers* **2**: 15082.

Grunt S, Becher JG, Vermeulen RJ (2011) Long-term outcome and adverse effects of selective dorsal rhizotomy in children with cerebral palsy: a systematic review. *Dev Med Child Neurol* **53**: 490–498.

Haberfehlner H, Goudriaan M, Bonouvrie LA et al. (2020) Instrumented assessment of motor function in dyskinetic cerebral palsy: A systematic review. *J NeuroEng Rehab* **17**.

Hanna SE, Bartlett DJ, Rivard LM, Russell DJ (2008) Reference curves for the Gross Motor Function Measure: percentiles for clinical description and tracking over time among children with cerebral palsy. *Phys Ther* **88**: 596–607.

Harvey AR, Baker LB, Reddihough DS, Scheinberg A, Williams K (2018) Trihexyphenidyl for dystonia in cerebral palsy. *Cochrane Database Syst Rev* **5**: CD012430.

Hemingway C, McGrogan J, Freeman JM (2001) Energy requirements of spasticity. *Dev Med Child Neurol* **43**: 277–278.

Himmelmann K, McManus V, Hagberg G, Uvebrant P, Krageloh-Mann I, Cans C (2009) Dyskinetic cerebral palsy in Europe: trends in prevalence and severity. *Arch Dis Child* **94**: 921–926.

Hoque M, Borich M, Sabatier M, Backus D, Kesar T (2019) Effects of downslope walking on Soleus H-reflexes and walking function in individuals with multiple sclerosis: A preliminary study. *NeuroRehabilitation* **44**: 587–597.

Hoque MM, Ardizzone MA, Sabatier M, Borich MR, Kesar TM (2018a) Longer Duration of Downslope Treadmill Walking Induces Depression of H-Reflexes Measured during Standing and Walking. *Neurology* **10**: 761–770.

Hoque MM, Sabatier MJ, Borich M, Kesar T, Backus D (2018b) The Short-Term Effect of Slope Walking on Soleus H-Reflexes in People with Multiple Sclerosis. *Neuroscience* **391**: 73–80.

Hosl M, Bohm H, Eck J, Doderlein L, Arampatzis A (2018) Effects of backward-downhill treadmill training versus manual static plantarflexor stretching on muscle-joint pathology and function in children with spastic Cerebral Palsy. *Gait Posture* **65**: 121–128.

Koy A, Hellmich M, Pauls KA et al. (2013) Effects of deep brain stimulation in dyskinetic cerebral palsy: a meta-analysis. *Mov Disord* **28**: 647–654.

Liang JN, Lee YJ, Akoopie E, Kleven BC, Koch T, Ho KY (2019) Impaired H-Reflex Adaptations Following Slope Walking in Individuals With Post-stroke Hemiparesis. *Front Physiol* **10**: 1232.

Linden O, Hagglund G, Rodby-Bousquet E, Wagner P (2019) The development of spasticity with age in 4,162 children with cerebral palsy: a register-based prospective cohort study. *Acta Ortho* **90**: 286–291.

Lorentzen J, Kirk H, Fernandez-Lago H et al. (2017) Treadmill training with an incline reduces ankle joint stiffness and improves active range of movement during gait in adults with cerebral palsy. *Disabil Rehabil* **39**: 987–993.

McLaughlin J, Bjornson K, Temkin N et al. (2002) Selective dorsal rhizotomy: meta-analysis of three randomized controlled trials. *Dev Med Child Neurol* **44**: 17–25.

Minamoto VB, Suzuki KP, Bremner SN, Lieber RL, Ward SR (2015) Dramatic changes in muscle contractile and structural properties after 2 botulinum toxin injections. *Muscle Nerve* **52**: 649–657.

Monbaliu E, Himmelmann K, Lin JP et al. (2012) The Dyskinesia Impairment Scale: a new instrument to measure dystonia and choreoathetosis in dyskinetic cerebral palsy. *Dev Med Child Neurol* **54**: 278–283.

Monbaliu E, Himmelmann K, Lin JP et al. (2017) Clinical presentation and management of dyskinetic cerebral palsy. *Lancet Neurol* **16**: 741–749.

Mrachacz-Kersting N, Kersting UG, de Brito Silva P et al. (2019) Acquisition of a simple motor skill: task-dependent adaptation and long-term changes in the human soleus stretch reflex. *J Neurophysiol* **122**: 435–446.

Multani I, Manji J, Hastings-Ison T, Khot A, Graham K (2019) Botulinum Toxin in the Management of Children with Cerebral Palsy. *Paediatr Drugs* **21**: 261–281.

Munger ME, Aldahondo N, Krach LE, Novacheck TF, Schwartz MH (2017). Long-term outcomes after selective dorsal rhizotomy: a retrospective matched cohort study. *Dev Med Child Neurol* **59**: 1196–1203.

Novak I, McIntyre S, Morgan C et al. (2013) A systematic review of interventions for children with cerebral palsy: state of the evidence. *Dev Med Child Neurol* **55**: 885–910.

Ostojic K, Paget SP, Morrow AM (2019) Management of pain in children and adolescents with cerebral palsy: a systematic review. *Dev Med Child Neurol* **61**: 315–321.

Parent A, Raison M, Pouliot-Laforte A, Marois P, Maltais DB, Ballaz L (2016) Impact of a short walking exercise on gait kinematics in children with cerebral palsy who walk in a crouch gait. *Clin Biomech (Bristol, Avon)* **34**: 18–21.

Reddihough DS, King JA, Coleman GJ et al. (2002) Functional outcome of botulinum toxin A injections to the lower limbs in cerebral palsy. *Dev Med Child Neurol* **44**: 820–827.

Reid S, Hamer P, Alderson J, Lloyd D (2010) Neuromuscular adaptations to eccentric strength training in children and adolescents with cerebral palsy. *Dev Med Child Neurol* **52**: 358–363.

Rice J, Skuza P, Baker F, Russo R, Fehlings D (2017) Identification and measurement of dystonia in cerebral palsy. *Dev Med Child Neurol* **59**: 1249–1255.

Romeiser Logan L, Hickman R, Harris S, Heriza C (2008) Single-subject research design: Recommendations for levels of evidence and quality rating. *Developmental medicine and child neurology* **50**: 99–103.

Roubertie A, Mariani LL, Fernandez-Alvarez E, Doummar D, Roze E (2012) Treatment for dystonia in childhood. *Eur J Neurol* **19**: 1292–1299.

Sabatier MJ, Wedewer W, Barton B, Henderson E, Murphy JT, Ou K (2015) Slope walking causes short-term changes in soleus H-reflex excitability. *Physiol Rep* **3**.

Saxena S, Kumaran S, Rao BK (2016) Energy expenditure during standing in children with cerebral palsy: A brief report1. *J Pediatr Rehabil Med* **9**: 241–245.

Schasfoort F, Pangalila R, Sneekes EM et al. (2018) Intramuscular botulinum toxin prior to comprehensive rehabilitation has no added value for improving motor impairments, gait kinematics and goal attainment in walking children with spastic cerebral palsy. *J Rehabil Med* **50**: 732–742.

Sloot LH, van den Noort JC, van der Krogt MM, Bruijn SM, Harlaar J (2015) Can Treadmill Perturbations Evoke Stretch Reflexes in the Calf Muscles? *PLoS One* **10**: e0144815.

Surveillance of Cerebral Palsy in Europe (2000) Surveillance of cerebral palsy in Europe: a collaboration of cerebral palsy surveys and registers. *Dev Med Child Neurol* **42**: 816-824.

Tedroff K (2009) *Children with spastic cerebral palsy: aspects of muscle activity and botulinum toxin A treatment.* Stockholm: Department of woman and child health, Karolinska institutet.

Tedroff K, Befrits G, Tedroff CJ, Gantelius S (2018) To switch from Botox to Dysport in children with CP, a real world, dose conversion, cost-effectiveness study. *Eur J Paediatr Neurol* **22**: 412–418.

Tedroff K, Gyllensvard M, Lowing K (2019a) Prevalence, identification, and interference of pain in young children with cerebral palsy: a population-based study. *Disabil Rehabil* 1–7.

Tedroff K, Hagglund G, Miller F (2019b) Long-term effects of selective dorsal rhizotomy in children with cerebral palsy: a systematic review. *Dev Med Child Neurol* **62**: 554–562.

Tervo RC, Symons F, Stout J, Novacheck T (2006) Parental report of pain and associated limitations in ambulatory children with cerebral palsy. *Arch Phys Med Rehabil* **87**: 928–934.

Thomason P, Tan A, Donnan A, Rodda J, Graham HK, Narayanan U (2018) The Gait Outcomes Assessment List (GOAL): validation of a new assessment of gait function for children with cerebral palsy. *Dev Med Child Neurol* **60**: 618–623.

Thompson AK, Pomerantz FR, Wolpaw JR (2013) Operant conditioning of a spinal reflex can improve locomotion after spinal cord injury in humans. *J Neurosci* **33**: 2365–2375.

Thompson AK, Wolpaw JR (2019) H-reflex conditioning during locomotion in people with spinal cord injury. *J Physiol.* **10**: 1113

Turner-Stokes L (2009) Goal attainment scaling (GAS) in rehabilitation: a practical guide. *Clin Rehabil* **23**: 362–370.

Tustin K, Elze MC, Lumsden DE, Gimeno H, Kaminska M, Lin JP (2019) Gross motor function outcomes following deep brain stimulation for childhood-onset dystonia: A descriptive report. *Eur J Paediatr Neurol* **23**: 473–483.

van de Pol LA, Vermeulen RJ, van't Westende C et al. (2018) Risk Factors for Dystonia after Selective Dorsal Rhizotomy in Nonwalking Children and Adolescents with Bilateral Spasticity. *Neuropediatrics* **49**: 44–50.

van der Krogt MM, Doorenbosch CA, Becher JG, Harlaar J (2009a) Walking speed modifies spasticity effects in gastrocnemius and soleus in cerebral palsy gait. *Clin Biomech (Bristol, Avon)* **24**: 422–428.

van der Krogt MM, Doorenbosch CA, Harlaar J (2009b) The effect of walking speed on hamstrings length and lengthening velocity in children with spastic cerebral palsy. *Gait Posture* **29**: 640–644.

van Vulpen LF, de Groot S, Rameckers E, Becher JG, Dallmeijer AJ (2017) Improved Walking Capacity and Muscle Strength After Functional Power-Training in Young Children With Cerebral Palsy. *Neurorehabil Neural Repair* **31**: 827–841.

van Vulpen LF, de Groot S, Rameckers EA, Becher JG, Dallmeijer AJ (2018) Improved parent-reported mobility and achievement of individual goals on activity and participation level after functional power-training in young children with cerebral palsy: a double-baseline controlled trial. *Eur J Phys Rehabil Med* **54**: 730–737.

Vidailhet M, Vercueil L, Houeto JL et al.; French SPIDY Study Group (2007) Bilateral, pallidal, deep-brain stimulation in primary generalised dystonia: a prospective 3 year follow-up study. *Lancet Neurol* **6**: 223–229.

Ward SR, Minamoto VB, Suzuki KP, Hulst JB, Bremner SN, Lieber RL (2018) Recovery of rat muscle size but not function more than 1 year after a single botulinum toxin injection. *Muscle Nerve* **57**: 435–441.

Motor Control
Missing Links Between Neurological Injury and Movement that Limit Care and Function

Katherine M Steele and Warren A Marks

KEY POINTS

- Every brain injury is unique, such that each individual must develop a unique motor control strategy to move and explore their world.
- Motor control is associated with function and treatment outcomes.
- Current treatments, including therapy and surgical interventions, produce minimal changes in motor control.

OPPORTUNITIES

- Advances in neural imaging and stimulation can help link neurological injury with walking function.
- Biofeedback training may provide a platform to evaluate and accelerate motor learning.
- Early detection and monitoring can enhance our knowledge of motor control development.

Motor control is broadly defined as the strategies we use to recruit and coordinate our muscles to produce movement (Sherrington 1910; Perry 1969; Pearson 1976; Ting et al. 2015). It represents the confluence of numerous complex systems: motor planning, execution, feedback processing, adaptation, and learning. For individuals with cerebral palsy (CP), a brain injury can affect some or all of these processes, as well as introduce additional impairments – like spasticity or ataxia – that must be integrated into a control strategy. Every brain injury is unique; as well as the subsequent rewiring, learning, and development that occurs after the initial insult (Ferriero 2004). Two individuals who have seemingly similar injuries (e.g. periventricular leukomalacia) can develop very different motor control strategies and function (Yokochi

2001). This complexity makes evaluating, understanding, and treating gait impairments among people with CP incredibly challenging. Although we often refer to CP as an 'umbrella term' that captures several distinct neurological injuries, we are increasingly recognizing that the processes that influence motor learning and activity after the initial injury strongly influence the spectrum of function observed later in life. By understanding these processes, we can help identify activities or interventions that can support neuroplasticity and enhance long-term function.

While we have extensive tools for evaluating musculoskeletal impairments in CP, evaluating motor control is much more difficult. We can use motor outputs to attempt to decode underlying motor control strategies, such as evaluating an individual's ability to isolate movement of individual joints (e.g. Selective Control Assessment of the Lower Extremity [SCALE]), monitoring muscle activity with electromyography (EMG) recordings, or comparing instrumented spasticity assessments to muscle function during gait (Perry and Hoffer 1977; Desloovere et al. 2006; Fowler et al. 2010; Bar-On et al. 2013; Steele et al. 2015; Steele et al. 2019). However, these examinations only let us observe the net output of the motor system. This net output includes an individual's motor plan, based on years of motor learning, as well as their ability to execute this plan, integrate real-time feedback from sensory signals, and adapt to their current environment. Separating where in this pipeline impairments occur is nearly impossible. Two individuals may demonstrate poor selective motor control during physical exam, but the root cause could be very different. One individual may have decreased inhibition that causes excessive activation of other muscles, while the other may have excessive sensory feedback that triggers other muscles to activate (Nashner et al. 1983; Leonard et al. 1990). Decoding and understanding the interplay between these systems is critical to effectively design treatments that can improve gait and function for people with CP.

Despite the limitations of our current methods, we know that an individual's motor control is closely related to their function and treatment outcomes (Chambers et al. 1998; Damiano et al. 2000; Fowler and Goldberg 2009; Schwartz et al. 2016, Shuman et al. 2018). The most common measures used clinically to evaluate motor control are physical exam measurements and EMG recordings. From physical exam, we evaluate an individual's ability to isolate and selectively move each joint (e.g. SCALE), as well as test for spasticity, dystonia, and other signs of hyper- or hypotonicity (see Chapter 5). The EMG recordings from gait analysis can be used to examine the activity of individual muscles (e.g. excessive rectus femoris activity contributing to stiff-knee gait), quantify sequential contraction of antagonist muscle groups, and evaluate overall complexity of control during gait from synergy analyses (Ikeda et al. 1998; Reinbolt et al. 2008; Shuman et al. 2017). These exams start to reveal an individual's control strategy that can be used to detangle the factors contributing to impaired movement. Individuals who have motor control more similar to typically developing peers have better function and greater improvements in walking function after a broad array of treatments, including botulinum neurotoxin A injections, selective dorsal rhizotomy, and orthopedic surgery (Hayek et al. 2010; Schwartz et al. 2016; Shuman et al. 2018). This makes sense, as individuals with 'better' motor control will have greater capacity to utilize changes due to orthopedic surgery or intensive rehabilitation to improve gait. Unfortunately, we also see evidence that motor control is very challenging to change for people with CP (Patikas et al. 2007; Shuman et al. 2019). Even after surgical interventions that include intensive inpatient rehabilitation, there are minimal changes in motor control after treatment.

Given the importance of motor control to function, there are several critical gaps we need to fill to advance care and quality of life for people with CP. The following section outlines three gaps that severely limit our current care and treatment: (1) understanding the link between neurology and function, (2) evaluating the development of motor control, and (3) examining the plasticity of motor control for people with CP. Filling these gaps will provide important knowledge to guide future research and care for people with CP.

CRITICAL GAPS

Linking Neurology and Function

CP is a movement disorder caused by abnormal development or injury to the developing brain (Rosenbaum 2007). The subsequent care, cultural practices, activities, and positions the infant encounters further impacts the neurological circuits that develop and support movement (Adolph and Hoch 2019). Given the broad array of factors that impact early neurological development, predicting and guiding an individual's development with current tools is nearly impossible. While imaging techniques like ultrasound and magnetic resonance imaging (MRI) have demonstrated modest correlations with function, they largely capture volumetric defects or deviations from typically-developing norms that are challenging to tie to function (Krishnan et al. 2007; Rose et al. 2007; Zhou et al. 2017). We need new tools to evaluate and monitor these circuits and link them to motor function.

This need is rooted in not just understanding the initial neural insult, but also the development and function of neural circuits that support function. To tackle this challenge, we will need better resolution for evaluating the brain, spinal cord, and peripheral nervous system, as well as the ability to dynamically monitor and probe the function of these circuits during tasks of daily living. Advances in imaging and stimulation have recently shown promise for linking neurophysiology with upper extremity function for people with CP. By combining diffusion tensor imaging that can elucidate neural connectivity, with functional stimulation techniques like transcranial magnetic stimulation, researchers have been able to demonstrate important differences in neural circuits that impact arm and hand function (Friel et al. 2014; Bleyenheuft et al. 2015; Schertz et al. 2016; Robert et al. 2019). Unfortunately, these methods are much more challenging to apply to the lower extremity. While the upper-extremities have large and easily accessible representations within the motor and sensory cortices, lower extremity circuitry is represented by much smaller areas that are deep within the longitudinal fissure. This makes evaluating neural connections and stimulating the brain to evaluate impacts on movement more difficult for the lower extremity. Spinal circuits (e.g. central pattern generators and reflex loops) also play a much larger role in lower extremity function (Duysens and Van de Crommert 1998; Ivanenko et al. 2006), yet evaluating the function of these circuits and the impact of cortical control is challenging.

Beyond neural circuitry, linking neurology to function also requires new methods that can distinguish and probe the constituent components that influence motor control. In particular, our understanding of motor planning, feedback processing, and learning among people with CP is extremely limited (Jongbloed-Pereboom et al. 2012; Kurz et al. 2014a). We currently lack methods to clinically evaluate whether impaired movement is due to poor motor planning or flawed execution of an accurate motor plan. Similarly, evaluating whether and how sensory feedback influences movement, or whether errors in an individual's sensory feedback contributes to impaired movement remains unknown (Bumin and Kayihan 2001). While we can observe changes in function after an intervention, which might be indicative of motor learning, we struggle to understand whether an individual's response is indicative of motor learning, hindered by deficits in motor learning, or due to other effects of the intervention (e.g. strengthening muscles). Improving gait for people with CP requires new tools and techniques that can probe individual differences in neural circuitry and leverage these differences to guide treatment.

Tracking Development

Extensive prior research has monitored the development of gait among children with typical development. These studies demonstrate the importance of play and exploration during the development of motor milestones (Pellegrini and Smith 1998; Bornstein et al. 2013; Adolph and Franchak 2017). They also illustrate the wide range of strategies that typically developing children test and try during development. While the sitting, crawling, and walking strategies that children adopt vary greatly between individuals, they largely converge by 5 years of age to a highly-efficient, stereotypical walking pattern (Ivanenko et al. 2007; Adolph et al. 2011; Karasik et al. 2011). When examining motor control, researchers have used EMG recordings to evaluate how infants and toddlers recruit and coordinate their muscles. When starting to stand and walk, toddlers use very simple motor control strategies, such as basic flexion and extension synergies, that are thought to reflect reliance on spinal circuits like central pattern generators (Cooke and Thelen 1987; Yang et al. 2004; Ivanenko et al. 2013). Their motor control at this stage is very similar to EMG recordings during rhythmic stepping in young infants (Forssberg 1985). As they play and explore, motor control complexity increases. Toddlers learn through experience to utilize corticospinal pathways and integrate sensory feedback to create more flexible and efficient movement patterns. By grade school, motor control and gait patterns largely resemble those used by adults (Dominici et al. 2011).

Children with CP often have delayed movement, less daily movement, and less exploration that impacts this development (Leonard et al. 1991; Bjornson et al. 2014). If we examine motor control during gait of children with CP from clinical gait analyses (typically after 5–7 years of age), it closely resembles the early motor control strategies used by typically developing toddlers (Steele et al. 2015). Simplified motor control, with reliance on flexion and extension synergies, is common among children with CP. These motor control strategies are hypothesized to reflect continued reliance on spinal circuits, which impair movement and hinder more complex movements (e.g. climbing stairs or responding to a perturbation) that require greater reliance on corticospinal circuits (Johnson et al. 1997).

Monitoring early development of motor control, similar to prior work with typically developing children (Dominici et al. 2011), would provide a foundation for understanding impaired motor control and movement. Tracking the trajectory of development would demonstrate the range of motor control strategies adopted by children with CP and how they are influenced by and impact function. For example, examining how early movement strategies, exploration, or interventions like orthoses or walkers impact motor control has important implications for designing and prescribing early intervention programs. Determining when and how motor control strategies deviate from typically developing peers may also indicate critical time periods or motor milestones that can amplify the impact of interventions or prevent the need for more intensive treatment later in life. While early diagnosis and monitoring of children with CP remains challenging (Novak et al. 2017), this represents an important priority to advance care and function for people with CP.

Evaluating Neuroplasticity

Neuroplasticity refers to the ability of the nervous system to create and rewire connections. The neuroplasticity of motor systems in CP from childhood through adulthood is poorly understood. For many years, it was often assumed that individuals with CP had minimal neuroplasticity, but rather clinicians and therapists had to work with an individual's unique neural capacity. This led to clinical standards like insurance not supporting EMG recordings during gait analysis after surgical interventions, assuming there would be no changes in motor control, and few treatment options for teens and adults with CP. However, recent evidence in people with CP and typically developing adults suggests that the nervous system has greater capacity for neuroplasticity throughout the lifespan than previously thought (Valkanova et al. 2014; McDonnell et al. 2015; Porto et al. 2015).

Evaluating the potential for neuroplasticity and approaches that maximize neuroplasticity to improve function represent important areas of research in CP. For gait, the potential for neuroplasticity is still unclear. Prior research has suggested that motor control is very challenging to change in CP. There are minimal changes in motor control during gait after botulinum neurotoxin A injections, orthopedic surgery, or selective dorsal rhizotomy, even though many of these procedures include intensive, inpatient rehabilitation (Patikas et al. 2007; Shuman et al. 2019). Similarly, biofeedback training programs that target specific gait deficits (e.g. increase knee extension or step length) can improve walking function, but demonstrate minimal changes in motor control (Booth et al. 2019b). However, none of these interventions directly target motor control during walking or other tasks of daily living. Recent evidence of neuroplasticity after upper extremity training, including adults with CP, suggests that appropriately designed and customized training can enhance neuroplasticity (Phillips 2007; Lee et al. 2014; Reid et al. 2015; Friel et al. 2017). Overall, we are still optimistic that targeted interventions can induce meaningful neuroplasticity for people with CP.

Determining the potential for neuroplasticity is critically important. As noted above, individuals with CP who have poor motor control have worse function and worse outcomes after common treatments. If motor control is not plastic, we need to determine alternative strategies for improving function for people with CP who have poor motor control. An individual's unique motor control strategy could be used to evaluate expected treatment outcomes or serve as a constraint when designing new surgeries or assistive technologies. If motor control is plastic, this opens the door to new treatment strategies that can target an individual's unique needs. Individuals with poor motor control could undergo intensive rehabilitation before surgical interventions to improve their motor control and expected treatment outcomes. Targeted interventions that improve motor control and function could also prevent secondary musculoskeletal deformities and the need for invasive treatments. Understanding neuroplasticity also supports our need to better understand early development of motor control and motor learning. Together, these gaps represent challenging but pressing needs for our community.

OPPORTUNITIES

There are numerous technical and clinical advancements that can help accelerate research to fill these gaps. In particular, advances in neuroimaging and stimulation provide new tools that can improve the precision, breadth, and clinical translation of our work. Functional and anatomical neuroimaging methods, from ultrasound to functional MRI, are expanding our ability to evaluate each unique brain injury. As discussed above, these methods are largely being used to examine upper extremity function, due to challenges in deploying these techniques for lower extremity cortical areas, but we are confident that the precision and accuracy of these systems will continue to improve. Non-invasive methods like electroencephalography that can monitor cortical activity during dynamic tasks are also improving in their ability to provide meaningful and clinically relevant measures during gait (Kulak and Sobaniec 2005; Rigoldi et al. 2012; Kurz et al. 2014b). There are also a broad range of stimulation techniques, such as transcranial magnetic stimulation or transcranial direct current stimulation, that can be used to stimulate neural circuits (Bleyenheuft et al. 2015; Fleming et al. 2018; Hamilton et al. 2018). Researchers are exploring the use of these techniques to understand neural connectivity, by stimulating a region and observing the response, and as potential therapeutic techniques to induce neuroplasticity or target specific pathways. There are still numerous challenges to overcome in deploying and interpreting the results of these methods, but they represent exciting opportunities to support our understanding of neurophysiology in CP.

Biofeedback training refers to monitoring signals from an individual's body and providing feedback from those signals to inform training (Huang et al. 2006). The signals can capture many facets of an individual's movement: temporospatial parameters like walking speed or step length, kinematic measures like hip or knee extension, measures of muscle activity from EMG recordings, or even neurophysiological recordings from the modalities discussed above. Feedback can also be provided in many different forms, such as visual displays, audio ques, or vibration. From sports to daily activity, properly designed biofeedback training has been shown to be effective at improving performance (Vernon 2005). Biofeedback training also has a rich history in clinical use, especially among individuals with neurological injuries like CP or stroke (Basmajian et al. 1977; Wolf et al. 1980; Seeger and Caudrey 1983; Cozean et al. 1988; Wolf 1990; Bradley et al. 1998; Dursun et al. 2004; Jonsdottir et al. 2007; Nelson 2007; Bloom et al. 2010; Yoo et al. 2017; Booth et al. 2019a). While these techniques have shown promise for improving function, the technology required has limited clinical translation. Further, most techniques have not targeted motor control and have shown minimal impact on motor control during gait (Booth et al. 2019b). In the past decade, the tools to monitor movement and provide feedback have proliferated and now provide compelling platforms to test and deploy biofeedback training (Shull et al. 2014). In the clinic, monitoring EMG or other neural signals in real-time to provide feedback is now feasible. Outside of the clinic, wearable technology that includes measures of muscle activity and movement (i.e. inertial measurement units) opens the door to more intensive training, with greater practice and feedback during activities of daily living. While research is still required to determine the optimal methods for deploying these techniques in the clinic and community, they open the door to new strategies to monitor and improve motor control for people with CP.

CONCLUSION

Motor control is complex. Brain injuries are unique. These facts hinder our ability to evaluate, treat, and improve quality of life for people with CP. Multidisciplinary collaborations between neuroscientists, engineers, and clinicians will be required to provide the knowledge and techniques to fill these critical gaps. Understanding the link between neurophysiology and function, and leveraging this knowledge to improve care offers exciting pathways that may transform how we evaluate and treat gait impairments for people with CP.

5-YEAR PRIORITIES

- **Monitor development:** measure the development of motor control during the first 5 years of life for children with CP and compare to typically developing peers.
- **Evaluate plasticity:** evaluate motor control using multiple modalities at multiple time points before and after current interventions.
- **Target plasticity:** determine when and whether novel interventions, such as biofeedback training or exoskeletons that specifically target muscle activity, can induce changes in an individual's motor control during walking.

FUTURE NEEDS

- **Precision for the lower extremity:** neural circuits, both in the cortex and spinal cord, that dictate lower extremity function are challenging to access. New strategies are needed to easily and reliably access and assess these circuits.
- **Differentiate motor learning and planning:** motor control represents the net effect of motor planning, execution, feedback integration, learning, and other processes. New tools are needed to differentiate and examine the interplay of these processes and impairments in specific processes for people with CP.

- **Sensory feedback:** brain injury impacts the motor and sensory cortices, yet we focus most of our attention on motor impairments. The interplay of motor and sensory impairments on function and treatment outcomes needs greater attention.
- **Inhibition:** many of our tools (e.g. EMG, transcranial magnetic stimulation, motion analysis) provide a measure of the net activation of our motor system. Quantifying and understanding the impact of impaired inhibition is an important area for future research.

REFERENCES

Adolph KE, Berger SE, Leo AJ (2011) Developmental continuity? Crawling, cruising, and walking. *Dev Sci* **14**: 306–318.

Adolph KE, Franchak JM (2017) The development of motor behavior. *Wiley Interdiscip Rev Cogn Sci* **8**: 1–2.

Adolph KE & Hoch JE (2019) Motor Development: Embodied, Embedded, Enculturated, and Enabling. *Annual review of psychology* **70**: 141–164.

Bar-On L, Aertbeliën E, Wambacq H et al. (2013) A clinical measurement to quantify spasticity in children with cerebral palsy by integration of multidimensional signals. *Gait Posture* **38**: 141–147.

Basmajian JV, Regenos EM, Baker MP (1977) Rehabilitating stroke patients with biofeedback. *Geriatrics* **32**: 85–88.

Bjornson KF, Zhou C, Stevenson R, Christakis D, Song K (2014) Walking activity patterns in youth with cerebral palsy and youth developing typically. *Disabil Rehabil* **36**: 1279–1284.

Bleyenheuft Y, Dricot L, Gilis N et al. (2015) Capturing neuroplastic changes after bimanual intensive rehabilitation in children with unilateral spastic cerebral palsy: A combined DTI, TMS and fMRI pilot study. *Research in Developmental Disabilities* **43**: 136–149.

Bloom R, Przekop A, Sanger TD (2010) Prolonged electromyogram biofeedback improves upper extremity function in children with cerebral palsy. *Journal of Child Neurology* **25**: 1480–1484.

Booth AT, Buizer AI, Harlaar J, Steenbrink F, van der Krogt MM (2019a) Immediate effects of immersive biofeedback on gait in children with cerebral palsy. *Arch Phys Med Rehabil* **100**: 598–605.

Booth ATC, van der Krogt MM, Harlaar J, Dominici N, Buizer AI (2019b) Muscle synergies in response to biofeedback-driven gait adaptations in children with cerebral palsy. *Front Physiol* **10**: 1208.

Bornstein MH, Hahn CS, Suwalsky JT (2013) Physically developed and exploratory young infants contribute to their own long-term academic achievement. *Psychol Sci* **24**: 1906–1917.

Bradley L, Hart BB, Mandana S, Flowers K, Riches M, Sanderson P (1998) Electromyographic biofeedback for gait training after stroke. *Clin Rehabil* **12**: 11–22.

Bumin G, Kayihan H (2001) Effectiveness of two different sensory-integration programmes for children with spastic diplegic cerebral palsy. *Disabil Rehabil* **23**: 394-399.

Chambers H, Lauer A, Kaufman K, Cardelia JM, Sutherland D (1998) Prediction of outcome after rectus femoris surgery in cerebral palsy: the role of cocontraction of the rectus femoris and vastus lateralis. *Journal of Pediatric Orthopaedics* **18**: 703–711.

Clowry GJ (2007) The dependence of spinal cord development on corticospinal input and its significance in understanding and treating spastic cerebral palsy. *Neuroscience & Biobehavioral Reviews* **31**: 1114–1124.

Cooke DW, Thelen E (1987) Newborn stepping: a review of puzzling infant co-ordination. *Dev Med Child Neurol* **29**: 399–404.

Cozean CD, Pease WS, Hubbell SL (1988) Biofeedback and functional electric stimulation in stroke rehabilitation. *Arch Phys Med Rehabil* **69**: 401–405.

Damiano DL, Martellotta TL, Sullivan DJ, Granata KP, Abel MF (2000) Muscle force production and functional performance in spastic cerebral palsy: Relationship of cocontraction. *Archives of Physical Medicine and Rehabilitation* **81**: 895–900.

Desloovere K, Molenaers G, Feys H, Huenaerts C, Callewaert B, Van de Walle P (2006) Do dynamic and static clinical measurements correlate with gait analysis parameters in children with cerebral palsy? *Gait Posture* **24**: 302–313.

Dominici N, Ivanenko YP, Cappellini G et al. (2011) Locomotor primitives in newborn babies and their development. *Science* **334**: 997–999.

Dursun E, Dursun N, Alican D (2004) Effects of biofeedback treatment on gait in children with cerebral palsy. *Disabil Rehabil* **26**: 116–120.

Duysens J, Van de Crommert HW (1998) Neural control of locomotion; the central pattern generator from cats to humans. *Gait Posture* **7**: 131–141.

Eyre J (2007) Corticospinal tract development and its plasticity after perinatal injury. *Neuroscience & Biobehavioral Reviews* **31**: 1136–1149.

Ferriero DM (2004) Neonatal brain injury. *New england journal of medicine* **351**: 1985–1995.

Fleming MK, Theologis T, Buckingham R, Johansen-berg H (2018) Transcranial direct current stimulation for promoting motor function in cerebral palsy: A review. *J Neuroeng Rehabil* **15**: 121.

Forssberg H (1985) Ontogeny of human locomotor control I. Infant stepping, supported locomotion and transition to independent locomotion. *Exp Brain Res* **57**: 480–493.

Fowler EG, Goldberg EJ (2009) The effect of lower extremity selective voluntary motor control on interjoint coordination during gait in children with spastic diplegic cerebral palsy. *Gait Posture* **29**: 102-107.

Fowler EG, Staudt LA, Greenberg MB (2010) Lower-extremity selective voluntary motor control in patients with spastic cerebral palsy: Increased distal motor impairment. *Developmental Medicine & Child Neurology* **52**: 264–269.

Friel KM, Kuo HC, Carmel JB, Rowny SB, Gordon AM (2014) Improvements in hand function after intensive bimanual training are not associated with corticospinal tract dysgenesis in children with unilateral cerebral palsy. *Experimental Brain Research* **232**: 2001–2009.

Friel KM, Lee P, Soles LV et al. (2017) Combined transcranial direct current stimulation and robotic upper limb therapy improves upper limb function in an adult with cerebral palsy. *Neurorehabilitation* **41**: 41–50.

Hamilton A, Wakely L, Marquez J (2018) Transcranial direct-current stimulation on motor function in pediatric cerebral palsy: A systematic review. *Pediatr Phys Ther* **30**: 291–301.

Hayek S, Gershon A, Wientroub S, Yizhar Z (2010) The effect of injections of botulinum toxin type a combined with casting on the equinus gait of children with cerebral palsy. *The journal of bone and joint surgery. British Volume* **92**: 1152–1159.

Huang H, Wolf SL, He J (2006) Recent developments in biofeedback for neuromotor rehabilitation. *J NeuroEngineering Rehabil* **3**: 11.

Ikeda AJ, Abel MF, Granata KP, Damiano DL (1998) Quantification of cocontraction in spastic cerebral palsy. *Electromyography and Clinical Neurophysiology* **38**: 497–504.

Ivanenko YP, Dominici N, Cappellini G et al. (2013) Changes in the spinal segmental motor output for stepping during development from infant to adult. *J Neurosci* **33**: 3025–36a.

Ivanenko YP, Dominici N, Lacquaniti F (2007) Development of independent walking in toddlers. *Exerc Sport Sci Rev* **35**: 67–73.

Ivanenko YP, Poppele RE, Lacquaniti F (2006) Motor control programs and walking. *The Neuroscientist* **12**: 339–348.

Johnson DC, Damiano DL, Abel MF (1997) The evolution of gait in childhood and adolescent cerebral palsy. *J Pediatr Orthop* **17**: 392–396.

Jongbloed-Pereboom M, Janssen AJ, Steenbergen B, Nijhuis-van der sanden MW (2012) Motor learning and working memory in children born preterm: a systematic review. *Neurosci Biobehav Rev* **36**: 1314–1330.

Jonsdottir J, Cattaneo D, Regola A et al. (2007) Concepts of motor learning applied to a rehabilitation protocol using biofeedback to improve gait in a chronic stroke patient: an a-b system study with multiple gait analyses. *Neurorehabil Neural Repair* **21**: 190–194.

Karasik LB, Tamis-Lemonda CS, Adolph KE (2011) Transition from crawling to walking and infants' actions with objects and people. *Child Dev* **82**: 1199–1209.

Krishnan ML, Dyet LE, Boardman JP et al. (2007) Relationship between white matter apparent diffusion coefficients in preterm infants at term-equivalent age and developmental outcome at 2 years. *Pediatrics* **120**: e604–e609.

Kulak W, Sobaniec W (2005) Quantitative eeg analysis in children with hemiparetic cerebral palsy. *Neurorehabilitation* **20**: 75–84.

Kurz MJ, Becker KM, Heinrichs-Graham E, Wilson TW (2014a) Neurophysiological abnormalities in the sensorimotor cortices during the motor planning and movement execution stages of children with cerebral palsy. *Dev Med Child Neurol* **56**: 1072–1077.

Kurz MJ, Wilson TW, Arpin DJ (2014b) An fnirs exploratory investigation of the cortical activity during gait in children with spastic diplegic cerebral palsy. *Brain Dev* **36**: 870–877.

Lee DR, Kim YH, Kim DA et al. (2014) Innovative strength training-induced neuroplasticity and increased muscle size and strength in children with spastic cerebral palsy: an experimenter-blind case study--three-month follow-up. *Neurorehabilitation* **35**: 131–136.

Leonard CT, Hirschfeld H, Forssberg H (1991) The development of independent walking in children with cerebral palsy. *Dev Med Child Neurol* **33**: 567–577.

Leonard CT, Moritani T, Hirschfeld H, Forssberg, H (1990) Deficits in reciprocal inhibition of children with cerebral palsy as revealed by H reflex testing. *Developmental Medicine & Child Neurology* **32**: 974–984.

Martin JH, Friel KM, Salimi I, Chakrabarty S (2007) Activity-and use-dependent plasticity of the developing corticospinal system. *Neuroscience & Biobehavioral Reviews* **31**: 1125–1135.

Mcdonnell MN, Koblar S, Ward NS, Rothwell JC, Hordacre B, Ridding MC (2015) An investigation of cortical neuroplasticity following stroke in adults: is there evidence for a critical window for rehabilitation? *BMC Neurol* **15**: 109.

Nashner L, Shumway-Cook A, Marin O (1983) Stance posture control in select groups of children with cerebral palsy: deficits in sensory organization and muscular coordination. *Experimental Brain Research* **49**: 393–409.

Nelson LA (2007) The role of biofeedback in stroke rehabilitation: past and future directions. *Top Stroke Rehabil* **14**: 59–66.

Novak I, Morgan C, Adde L et al. (2017) Early, accurate diagnosis and early intervention in cerebral palsy: advances in diagnosis and treatment. *Jama Pediatr* **171**: 897–907.

Patikas D, Wolf S, Schuster W, Armbrust P, Dreher T, Döderlein L (2007) Electromyographic patterns in children with cerebral palsy: do they change after surgery? *Gait Posture* **26**: 362–371.

Pearson K (1976) The control of walking. *Scientific American* **235**: 72–87.

Pellegrini AD, Smith PK (1998) Physical activity play: the nature and function of a neglected aspect of playing. *Child Dev* **69**: 577–598.

Perry J (1969) The mechanics of walking in hemiplegia. *Clinical Orthopaedics and Related Research (1976–2007)* **63**: 23–31.

Perry J, Hoffer M (1977) Preoperative and postoperative dynamic electromyography as an aid in planning tendon transfers in children with cerebral palsy. *The Journal of Bone and Joint Surgery. American Volume* **59**: 531–537.

Phillips JP (2007) Neuroimaging in cerebral palsy: A clearer vision of neuroplasticity. *Neuropediatrics* **38**: 112–113.

Porto FH, Fox AM, Tusch ES, Sorond F, Mohammed AH, Daffner KR (2015) In vivo evidence for neuroplasticity in older adults. *Brain Res Bull* **114**: 56–61.

Reid LB, Rose SE, Boyd RN (2015) Rehabilitation and neuroplasticity in children with unilateral cerebral palsy. *Nat Rev Neurol* **11**: 390–400.

Reinbolt JA, Fox MD, Arnold AS, Óunpuu S, Delp SL (2008) Importance of preswing rectus femoris activity in stiff-knee gait. *Journal of Biomechanics* **41**: 2362–2369.

Rigoldi C, Molteni E, Rozbaczylo C et al. (2012) Movement analysis and eeg recordings in children with hemiplegic cerebral palsy. *Exp Brain Res* **223**: 517–524.

Robert MT, Gutterman J, Ferre CL et al. (2019) Improvements in upper extremity function in children with unilateral spastic cerebral palsy after intensive training correlates with interhemispheric connectivity. *bioRxiv* 609313.

Rose J, Mirmiran M, Butler EE et al. (2007) Neonatal microstructural development of the internal capsule on diffusion tensor imaging correlates with severity of gait and motor deficits. *Developmental Medicine & Child Neurology* **49**: 745–750.

Rosenbaum P, Paneth N, Leviton et al. (2007) A report: the definition and classification of cerebral palsy April 2006. *Dev Med Child Neurol Suppl* **109**: 8–14

Schertz M, Shiran SL, Myers V et al. (2016) Imaging predictors of improvement from a motor learning-based intervention for children with unilateral cerebral palsy. *Neurorehabil Neural Repair* **30**: 647–660.

Schwartz MH, Rozumalski A, Steele KM (2016) Dynamic motor control is associated with treatment outcomes for children with cerebral palsy. *Dev Med Child Neurol* **58**: 1139–1145.

Seeger BR, Caudrey DJ (1983) Biofeedback therapy to achieve symmetrical gait in children with hemiplegic cerebral palsy: long-term efficacy. *Arch Phys Med Rehabil* **64**: 160–162.

Sherrington C (1910) Remarks on the reflex mechanism of the step. *Brain* **33**: 1–25.

Shull PB, Jirattigalachote W, Hunt MA, Cutkosky MR, Delp SL (2014) Quantified self and human movement: A review on the clinical impact of wearable sensing and feedback for gait analysis and intervention. *Gait Posture* **40**: 11–19.

Shuman BR, Goudriaan M, Desloovere K, Schwartz MH, Steele KM (2018) Associations between muscle synergies and treatment outcomes in cerebral palsy are robust across clinical centers. *Arch Phys Med Rehabil* **99**: 2175–2182.

Shuman BR, Goudriaan M, Desloovere K, Schwartz MH, Steele KM (2019) Muscle synergies demonstrate only minimal changes after treatment in cerebral palsy. *J Neuroeng Rehabil* **16**: 46.

Shuman BR, Schwartz MH, Steele KM (2017) Electromyography data processing impacts muscle synergies during gait for unimpaired children and children with cerebral palsy. *Frontiers in Computational Neuroscience* **11**: 50.

Steele KM, Munger ME, Peters KM, Shuman BR, Schwartz MH (2019) Repeatability of electromyography recordings and muscle synergies during gait among children with cerebral palsy. *Gait Posture* **67**: 290–295.

Steele KM, Rozumalski A, Schwartz MH (2015) Muscle synergies and complexity of neuromuscular control during gait in cerebral palsy. *Developmental Medicine & Child Neurology* **57**: 1176–1182.

Ting LH, Chiel HJ, Trumbower RD et al. (2015) Neuromechanical principles underlying movement modularity and their implications for rehabilitation. *Neuron* **86**: 38–54.

Valkanova V, Eguia Rodriguez R, Ebmeier KP (2014) Mind over matter-What do we know about neuroplasticity in adults? *Int Psychogeriatr* **26**: 891–909.

Vernon DJ (2005) Can neurofeedback training enhance performance? An evaluation of the evidence with implications for future research. *Appl Psychophysiol Biofeedback* **30**: 347–364.

Wolf SL (1990) Use of biofeedback in the treatment of stroke patients. *Stroke* **21**: II22-II23

Wolf SL, Baker MP, Kelly JL (1980) Emg biofeedback in stroke: A 1-year follow-up on the effect of patient characteristics. *Arch Phys Med Rehabil* **61**: 351–355.

Yang JF, Lam T, Pang MY, Lamont E, Musselman K, Seinen E (2004) Infant stepping: a window to the behaviour of the human pattern generator for walking. *Can J Physiol Pharmacol* **82**: 662–674.

Yokochi K (2001) Gait patterns in children with spastic diplegia and periventricular leukomalacia. *Brain and Development* **23**: 34–37.

Yoo JW, Lee DR, Cha YJ, You SH (2017) Augmented effects of emg biofeedback interfaced with virtual reality on neuromuscular control and movement coordination during reaching in children with cerebral palsy. *Neurorehabilitation* **40**: 175–185.

Zhou J, Butler EE, Rose J (2017) Neurologic correlates of gait abnormalities in cerebral palsy: implications for treatment. *Frontiers in Human Neuroscience* **11**: 103.

The Muscle-Tendon Unit in Children with Cerebral Palsy and Pathophysiology of Muscle

Rick Lieber and Tim Theologis

KEY POINTS

- Lengthening and transfer are the two most common orthopaedic surgical interventions on muscle. However, length is not the only important problem: strength, tone, and neurological control need to be taken into account.
- Muscle-tendon unit lengthening causes significant and lasting weakness requiring prolonged rehabilitation. Increased sarcomere length in cerebral palsy (CP) muscle may be one of the underlying causes.
- A range of outcomes should be measured after orthopaedic interventions, and these have to represent the views of a wide range of stakeholders, including children, parents, and carers.

OPPORTUNITIES

- Develop modeling of muscle length and neurological control.
- Assess and compare rehabilitation regimes following multilevel surgery.
- Develop an agreed set of core outcomes to be consistently used following orthopaedic lower limb interventions for gait improvement in CP.

Mammalian skeletal muscles are remarkable machines that produce force and movement and have a design at the microscopic and macroscopic level that accomplishes this function (Enoka 1994; Lieber 2010). One of the most important functional properties of muscle is its isometric contractile properties (force developed at a fixed length) which can be both active (with muscle voluntarily activated or electrically stimulated) and passive (at rest or measured intraoperatively in an anesthetized patient [see Fig. 2 of Lieber et al. 2005]). Many surgical procedures are based on our general understanding of muscle properties reported in basic scientific studies. Perhaps the most complete presentations of surgical significance of muscle functional properties were presented by Dr Paul Brand in his classic monograph entitled, Clinical mechanics of the hand (Brand and Hollister 1993) and by Dr Jan Fridén in his monograph entitled, *Tendon transfers in reconstructive hand surgery* (2005). In this chapter, we will first review the basic properties of skeletal muscle and discuss their adaptation to cerebral palsy (CP). Then, we will describe the most common surgical procedures that alter the function of the muscle-tendon unit. Finally, we will suggest future directions that might improve our understanding of muscle-tendon units in CP as well as suggest potential treatments that might improve our patients' lives.

SKELETAL MUSCLE ISOMETRIC CONTRACTILE PROPERTIES

The isometric properties of muscle are determined by maximally stimulating a skeletal muscle at a series of discrete lengths and measuring the resulting tension generated by the muscle at each length. When maximum tetanic tension at each length is plotted against length, a nonlinear relationship such as that shown in Figure 7.1 is obtained. While a general description of this relationship was established early in the history of biology, the sarcomeric basis of the length-tension relationship was not elucidated until the sophisticated biomechanical experiments of the 1960s were performed (Edman 1966; Gordon, Huxley, and Julian 1966). These experiments defined the precise relationship between myofilament overlap within the sarcomere and tension generation, which we refer to today as the sarcomere length-tension relationship. In its most basic form, the length-tension relationship states that isometric tension generation in skeletal muscle is a direct function of the magnitude of overlap between actin and myosin filaments. Thus, when sarcomeres are either very long or very short, low isometric force is generated. However, at an 'optimal' length (where maximum interaction between myosin and actin filaments occurs), muscle generates its maximal force. As we will see, sarcomeres in muscle contractures are at abnormally long sarcomere lengths.

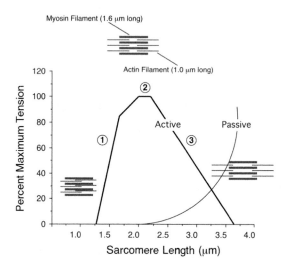

Figure 7.1 The sarcomere length-tension curve for frog skeletal muscle obtained using sequential isometric contractions in single muscle fibers. The figure shows the schematic arrangement of myofilaments in different regions of the length-tension curve. The dotted line represents passive muscle tension.

SKELETAL MUSCLE ARCHITECTURE

Skeletal muscle is not only highly organized to function at the microscopic sarcomere level, but the arrangement of the muscle fibers at the macroscopic level also demonstrates a striking degree of organization (Gans and Gaunt 1991; Lieber and Feidén 2000). In making comparisons among various muscles, certain factors such as fiber type distribution, capillary density, and connective tissue content are important, but there is no question that the most important factor that determines a muscle's active contractile properties is the muscle's architecture. Skeletal muscle architecture is defined as 'the arrangement of muscle fibers relative to the axis of force generation' (Gans and Gaunt 1991; Lieber and Feidén 2000). While muscle fibers (muscle cells) have a relatively consistent fiber diameter among muscles of vastly different sizes, the arrangements of these fibers can be quite different. The various types of arrangements are as numerous as the muscles themselves, but for convenience we often refer to three types of fiber architecture. Muscles with fibers that extend parallel to the muscle force-generating axis are termed parallel or longitudinally arranged muscles (Fig. 7.2a). Muscles with fibers that are oriented at a single angle relative to the force-generating axis are termed unipennate muscles (Fig. 7.2b). The angle between the fiber and the force-generating axis is relatively small, as can be appreciated by an intraoperative view of muscle, and this angle generally varies from 0° to 30° (Lieber, Fazeli, and Botte 1990; Lieber et al. 1992; Ward et al. 2009). It is obvious when dissecting muscle that most muscles fall into the final and most general category, multipennate muscles, which are composed of fibers that are oriented at several angles relative to the axis of force generation (Fig. 7.2c).

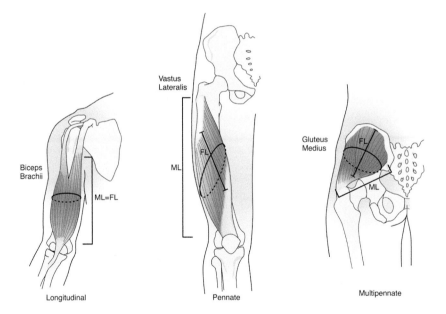

Figure 7.2 Generalized picture of muscle architecture types. Skeletal muscle fibers may be oriented parallel to the muscle's force-generating axis (*left*, known as longitudinal architecture), at a fixed angle relative to the force-generating axis (*middle*, known as pennate architecture), or at multiple angles relative to the force-generating axis (*right*, known as multipennate architecture). Each of these drawings represents an idealized view of muscle architecture and probably does not adequately describe any single muscle. ML, muscle length; FL, fiber length.

CONTRACTILE PROPERTIES OF MUSCLES WITH DIFFERENT ARCHITECTURES

An important functional consequence of muscle architecture is that the basic sarcomere properties are amplified by the number of sarcomeres arranged in series and in parallel to produce muscles with overall properties where peak force developed by the muscle is proportional to physiological cross-sectional area (number of sarcomeres in parallel [Powell et al. 1984; Winters et al. 2011]) and the excursion over which it acts is proportional to its muscle fiber length (number of sarcomeres in series [Bodine et al. 1982; Takahashi et al. 2012]). This point will be illustrated by comparing muscles of different architectures. Suppose that two muscles had identical fiber lengths and pennation angles, but one muscle had twice the mass (equivalent to saying that one muscle had twice the number of fibers and thus twice the physiological cross-sectional area). The functional difference between these two muscles is shown in Figure 7.3a: the muscle with twice the physiological cross-sectional area has a length-tension curve with the same shape but is amplified upward by a factor of two. Thus, the maximum tetanic tension (Po) of the larger muscle will be twice that of the smaller muscle. In the next example, consider the functional differences between two muscles with identical physiological cross-sectional areas and pennation angles but fiber lengths that differ by a factor of two. Figure 7.3b demonstrates that the effect increases muscle excursion. Peak absolute force of the length-tension curves is identical between muscles, but the absolute muscle active range is different. The architectural properties of most human upper extremity (Lieber, Fazeli, and Botte 1990; Lieber et al. 1992; Murray, Buchanan, and Delp 2000), lower extremity (Wickiewicz et al. 1983; Ward et al. 2009), and some axial muscles (Cleworth and Edman 1972; Ward et al. 2009; Brown et al. 2011) have been determined, and these parameters form the basis for our biomechanical understanding of muscle function and provide the core data for all musculoskeletal models used to predict human muscle function.

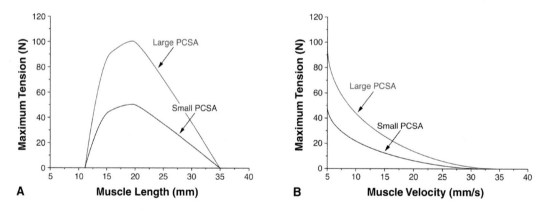

Figure 7.3 Schematic length-tension and force-velocity curves for muscle with different architectural properties. (a) Isometric length-tension curves for muscles with identical fiber but different cross-sectional areas. (b) Isometric length-tension curves for muscles with identical cross-sectional areas but different fibers.

INTRAOPERATIVE MEASUREMENT OF MUSCLE PROPERTIES

In an effort to improve our ability to perform surgical reconstruction of muscles, primarily in patients with tetraplegia, we have measured muscle properties during surgery. In March 1993, we performed laser diffraction in a human patient undergoing a hand surgery procedure. This laser diffraction method had been pioneered in 1972 by the Swedish physiologist Paul Edman (1972) and refined over the years by others (Rüdel and Zite 1980; Leung 1982; Lieber, Yeh, and Baskin 1984). The power of this method is that sarcomere length can be measured in living humans. Furthermore, this length can be checked, modeled, and compared to predictions in order to enable an understanding of human in vivo operating ranges (Burkholder and Lieber 2001). We used this method in a number of patients including those suffering from tennis elbow (Fridén and Lieber 1994; Ljung, Lieber, and Fridén 1999), peripheral nerve injury (Lieber and Fridén 1997), and spinal cord injury and used them to understand basic muscle design (Fridén and Lieber 2002), as well as to refine surgical procedures for specific patients (Lieber et al. 1996).

However, it is not an understatement to say that neither of us were prepared for the startling results obtained from measuring intraoperative sarcomere length in children with CP (Lieber and Fridén 2002). Because diffraction orders are spaced regularly with a stereotypical intensity profile (for example, see Fig. 1 of Lieber, Fazeli, and Botte 1990), when we inserted the laser into the contracture, it was immediately obvious that contracture sarcomeres were stretched to very long lengths (over $3.6\mu m$ with the wrist flexed, Fig. 7.4). Indeed, we performed a number of positive controls over the years to make sure that we were not being 'fooled' by some unknown alteration in sarcomere structure (Lieber, Loren, and Fridén 1994; Gokhin et al. 2009), nonrepresentative sarcomere lengths in a single muscle region (Ljung, Fridén, and Lieber 1999; Takahashi, Ward, and Liebber 2007), or overstretching a muscle fiber bundle with the laser device (Lieber, Loren, and Fridén 1994). We arrived at the very important conclusion that although muscle contractures represent shortened muscles, internal to the muscles are highly lengthened sarcomeres. It must be emphasized that this is a uniquely human condition. Experiments performed in the 1970s in mice, rats, rabbits, and cats clearly showed that, if a muscle is chronically stretched (typically by cast immobilization) the sarcomeres initially stretch and then the muscle mounts a tremendous synthesis of new sarcomeres to be added in series to the fibers, thus decreasing sarcomere length back to some 'set point' (Williams and Goldspink 1971; Tabary et al. 1972 Williams and Goldspink 1973). Chronically lengthened sarcomeres (perhaps in some patients for years) is simply not observed in any other mammalian system.

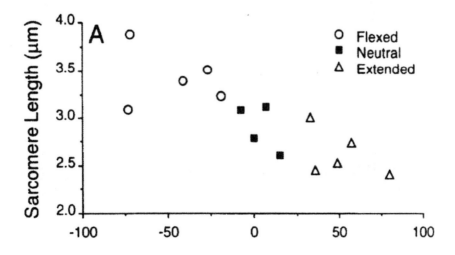

Figure 7.4 Sarcomere length vs wrist joint angle relationship determined for five patients. Negative angles represent wrist flexion relative to neutral, whereas positive angles represent wrist extension. One-way analysis of variance revealed a significant difference between wrist joint angles and sarcomere lengths in the three positions. o flexed angles; ■ neutral angles; Δ extended angles.

The functional implications of this finding, now confirmed for the soleus, gracilis, and semitendinosus muscles (Smith et al. 2011; Mathewson et al. 2015), are obvious based on the introductory material provided above. Longer sarcomeres produced lower forces compared to their shorter counterparts, and thus one reason muscles in CP are weaker than normal appears to be their lengthened sarcomeres. This also has surgical implications as tendon lengthening surgery is clearly a muscle shortening procedure. Based on this point alone, one would expect muscle force to increase with tendon lengthening procedures. However, as detailed in Chapter 8 of this book, tendon lengthening procedures tend to decrease muscle strength. Whether this is due to changes in neural activation or another as yet unidentified cause remains to be determined.

IN VITRO STUDIES OF HUMAN MUSCLE BIOPSIES

Small muscle biopsies were obtained during surgery to test the biomechanical properties of muscle fiber bundles and even single muscle cells. While we had suspected that cellular mechanical properties might be altered (since the children were so weak), we actually found cellular mechanical properties were relatively normal (Fridén and Lieber 2003). The main effect of CP was that the extracellular matrix (ECM) was hypertrophic and had altered properties (Lieber et al. 2003; Smith et al. 2012; Smith, Chambers, and Lieber 2013). In the upper extremity muscles, the ECM was surprisingly compliant, but in the lower extremity, the ECM was actually much stiffer compared to typically developing children. In fact, our biopsy biomechanical studies led us to examine muscle ECM which, as it turns out, was fairly understudied. We subsequently demonstrated a great deal of organization to the muscle ECM (Gillies and Lieber 2011; Gillies et al. 2017) and even biochemical changes in ECM (Smith et al. 2019) all of which combine to make a muscle that is much stiffer compared to normal muscles. Detailed morphometric measurement of these CP muscles showed a proliferation of fibroblasts that were probably responsible for deposition of much of this additional collagen.

DECREASED MUSCLE STEM CELLS IN CP

In spite of the altered ECM, we kept returning to this more profound phenotype of the very long sarcomeres in the CP muscle. The inability of contracture muscles to add sarcomeres prompted us to think about normal causes of muscle growth. During normal muscle fiber development, mononucleated myoblasts fuse to form multinucleated myotubes, which then fuse to form mature muscle fibers. Interestingly, some of the myoblast cells remain even into adulthood to act as 'stem cells' for the mature muscle fiber, which can be activated by injury, exercise, toxin injection, and other methods to proliferate and repair fibers or increase their size. We hypothesized that the satellite cell (SC) population of contractured muscle might be compromised. To test this hypothesis, we isolated satellite cells from contractures and found a 60% decrease in SC content (Fig. 7.5a). Because the ECM of these muscles was also altered, which could cause problems with SC isolation, we performed the same experiment using immunohistochemistry instead of cell isolation and achieved the same results (Fig. 7.5b). Thus, not only are muscle contractures composed of muscle with smaller fibers (see Fig. 4 of Dayanidhi et al. 2015), these fibers have fewer satellite cells. Why? At this point, we do not know. Clearly, the primary insult in CP is to the central nervous system, but a downstream effect is of satellite cell number in affected muscles to be decreased.

Decreased satellite cell number have also been observed in muscles from males with Duchenne muscular dystrophy (DMD) (Feige et al. 2018). In the case of DMD, the mechanism appears to be the repetitive degeneration and regeneration of muscle fibers in which the SCs are ultimately unable to replicate and repopulate the stem cell niche over time. Indeed, there are DMD therapies being developed in which SC turnover is directly addressed to enhance the longevity of muscle fibers.

INCREASED PROLIFERATION AND DECREASED MATURATION OF MUSCLE STEM CELLS IN CP

While we did not believe the same mechanism was at play in CP muscle (primarily because embryonic myosin heavy chain, the hallmark of regeneration, is not highly expressed in CP), we wanted to test the ability of SCs to proliferate and develop after removal from the body. In this way, we could test the basic biological properties of CP and typically developing children SCs in the same environment, without the confounding factor of hypertrophic ECM with an altered biochemical composition (Smith et al. 2019). Again, we were surprised at the result — CP SCs were hyperproliferative compared to typically developing children (Fig. 7.6a) but failed to develop large myotubes (Fig. 7.6b) and express proteins associated with myogenesis (see Fig. 4 of Domenighetti et al. 2018). As this phenotype was reminiscent of hyperproliferation observed in malignancies, we tested the hypothesis that these CP SCs had been epigenetically modified. While there is some evidence that CP has a slight genetic basis, it is relatively small compared to monogenetic muscle diseases such as DMD and spinal muscular atrophy. Since a major form of epigenetic regulation is to hypermethylated DNA promoter regions, we measured the methylation profile of DNA extracted from SCs. Global methylation was significantly greater in CP SCs compared to typically developing children SCs. Furthermore, when measuring specific genes involved in myogenesis, these were also hypermethylated. Of course, this finding does not prove that DNA hypermethylation causes muscle contractures in CP, but it provides a possible mechanism by which a central nervous system lesion could lead to a muscle contracture and several testable ideas in treatments.

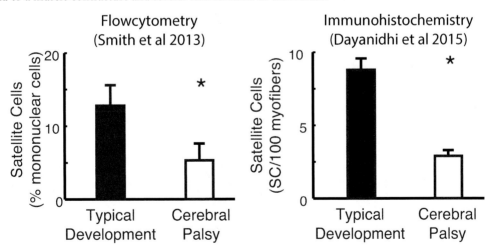

Figure 7.5 Satellite cells are muscle stem cells located in their niche between the blast lamina of the extracellular matrix and the sarcolemma of the myofibers. They are the source for myonuclei and indispensable for the growth and regeneration throughout life. In contractured muscles in children with CP, the satellite cell population is lower by 60 to 70% compared to children with typical development demonstrated using two different methods (flow cytometry and immunohistochemistry) in two different cohorts of children. Modified from Smith et al. (2013), Dayanidhi and Lieber (2014), and Dayanidhi et al. (2015).

PHARMACOLOGICAL 'RESCUE' OF MUSCLE STEM CELLS IN CP

An exciting experiment devised by my colleague Dr Andy Domenighetti was to test a U.S. Food and Drug Administration approved drug used for cancer on CP muscle cells. The drug, 5-azacytidine, is used to treat childhood blood cancer and has been sold in the United States for over 25 years under the trade name Vidaza. He treated CP SCs for 24-hours with 5-azacytidine and measured all of the standard parameters mentioned above. Importantly, 5-azacytidine 'rescued' the CP SCs from the maladaptive phenotype that had been observed and clearly restored their ability to differentiate and develop into mature muscle (Domenighetti 2018). This leads to the exciting possibility that 5-azacytidine treatment may serve as a therapeutic adjunct to surgery in the treatment of muscle contractures. If successful, we envision a multimodal rehabilitation strategy of early treatment with a cytidine analog in combination with physical therapy that may allow normalization of SC function and contractured muscles to grow, thus improving the child's strength and range of motion. This approach of combining surgical, rehabilitative, and pharmacological treatment may even lead to a completely new platform to perform drug screening on human tissues related to other types of debilitating muscle conditions (e.g. neuromuscular diseases).

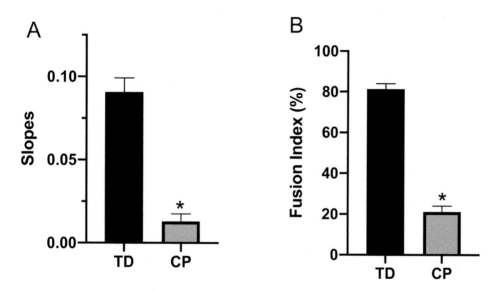

Figure 7.6 (A) Slopes of growth curves are used to quantify the rate of fusion and myotube formation over time: *CP vs typically developing children, $p<0.001$; one-way analysis of variance (ANOVA) ($n=8$/group). (B) Quantification of fusion index for CP and typically developing myoblasts. Quantification was performed after 42 hours of differentiation; *CP vs typically developing children, $p<0.001$; one-way ANOVA ($n=8$/group).

PATHOPHYSIOLOGY OF MUSCLE EFFECTS ON BIOMECHANICS, FUNCTION, AND QUALITY OF LIFE

One of the main clinical characteristics of cerebral palsy (CP) is expressed as a motor disorder affecting muscle function, most commonly in the form of spasticity or dystonia. Traditionally, the orthopaedic management of ambulant children with CP has involved muscle-tendon unit lengthening operations to address the apparently shortened units. Interventions were undertaken without full understanding of the biomechanics of gait and led to repeated surgeries and poor results, summarized by Dr Mercer Rang as the 'birthday syndrome' (Rang and Wenger 1993). With the evolution of gait analysis, our understanding of gait biomechanics improved, and the concept of single-event multilevel surgery (SEMLS) in ambulant children with CP evolved (Gage 2007). Although SEMLS also addressed bony deformity and lever-arm dysfunction, the muscle-tendon operations continued to form an integral part of the treatment and included lengthening, transfer of the attachment, and less frequently, shortening of units. As our understanding of muscle pathophysiology, neurological control, and function improves over time, surgical interventions on muscles are increasingly questioned. It is clear that our surgical interventions are imperfect and rather crude, considering the complexity of the problem they are addressing. In order to improve our surgery, we need to better understand pathophysiology and biomechanics of muscle function in CP. Moreover, we need to better understand the aims and goals of surgery, not only from the health professionals' perspective but also from the child and family's point of view.

ASSESSMENT OF MUSCLE

Clinical assessment of muscle forms part of the clinical examination in children with CP. Muscle atrophy may be visually evident. Palpation may reveal tenderness and pain. Range of motion of joints, particularly in combined joint positions, can give an indication of muscle length in static conditions (e.g. popliteal angle for the hamstrings). Depending on the velocity of joint movement, static and dynamic muscle contractures can be appreciated, and spasticity can be clinically assessed. Muscle strength can be assessed clinically or measured using dynamometers. Finally, selective motor control can be clinically assessed. More detailed studies of muscle, described by Dr Lieber earlier in this chapter, are based on detailed analysis of muscle biopsies or by intraoperative measurement of muscle properties.

Understanding how abnormalities identified during clinical examination translate into gait and motor function problems can be challenging. Static or dynamic examination of muscle length and the measurement of spasticity cannot reliably predict gait deviations (Rha et al. 2016; Choi et al. 2018). Differentiation between joint contracture, true muscle shortening, or dynamic shortening due to increased tone can also be challenging in a child with CP. Additional information on true versus dynamic muscle contracture can be obtained under anaesthesia. It is questionable, however, if this is indeed the ideal time to make rapid decisions on surgical interventions.

Although clinical examination largely focuses on the assessment of muscle length and contractures, muscle weakness is also an important characteristic of CP, which should be taken into account when considering orthopaedic interventions. Inadequate muscle development, incomplete activation, increased levels of antagonist coactivation, reduced physical activity levels, and the muscle structural changes discussed in Chapter 6, all contribute to the inadequate muscle strength observed clinically. It has been shown that muscle strength can be reliably and consistently measured in children with CP and that the reliability of the assessment improves with the use of handheld dynamometers and the standardization of patient positioning for measurement (Seniorou et al. 2007; Dallmeijer et al. 2011; Thompson et al. 2011).

As surgical lengthening of muscle further affects muscle strength (Seniorou et al. 2007), it is important to consider preoperative assessment of strength as part of the decision-making process.

Assessing the neurological control of muscle in a clinically meaningful way that would guide treatment decisions is particularly challenging. The assessment of spasticity and dystonia is covered in Chapter 5. From the surgical decision-making perspective, the clinical tools for the assessment of neurological muscle function are not sufficiently reliable and consistent (Bar-On et al. 2015; Meseguer-Henarejos et al. 2018). It is also difficult to predict muscle response to surgery and any changes to its neurological function that surgical interventions may introduce. Although there is some evidence that neurological muscle control remains unchanged after surgery (Schwartz, Rozumalski, and Steele 2016; Salami et al. 2018), there are exceptions to this rule, and surprises do occur (Piazza et al. 2003).

There is also evidence that spasticity and dystonia cause pain (Geister et al. 2014). Secondary musculoskeletal deformities may cause additional pain. It is possible that the level of pain in children with CP is underestimated. Pain should be formally assessed before and after any surgical interventions in children with ambulant CP, as it represents an important element of health-related quality of life.

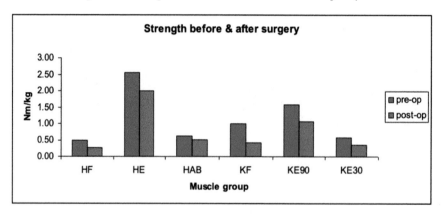

Figure 7.7 Loss of strength in lower limb muscles at 6 months following single event multi-level surgery (*n*=20).

HF: hip flexors (*sd*=0.14),
HE: hip extensors (*sd*=0.75),
HAB: hip abductors (*sd*=0.25),
KF: knee flexors (*sd*=0.21),
KE90: knee extensors at 90° flexion (*sd*=0.44),
KE30: knee extensors at 30° flexion (*sd*=0.19).

Instrumented assessment and modeling of muscle length and neurological control will be discussed in Chapter 8 of this book. Reliable muscle length assessment based on motion analysis kinematics would offer invaluable information when considering surgical interventions. Moreover, modeling of neurological control, spasticity, and weakness would offer a comprehensive preoperative assessment of pathological muscle function and allow realistic simulation of surgical interventions preoperatively. Currently, biomechanical modeling of muscle length and function is not reliable and accurate enough to be introduced into routine clinical practice. Functional muscle-tendon unit length at different points of the gait cycle can be inferred from analysis of the joint kinematic graphs. This is often used to confirm that muscle length is adequate and that lengthening is unnecessary. The hamstrings are a typical example where poor iatrogenic outcomes can often be avoided by using guidance from kinematics-derived muscle length and velocity.

However, individual anatomical variations can render the assumptions used by more complex musculo-skeletal modeling highly inaccurate, and tendon compliance, which allows muscle and tendon length to be dissociated, has not ever been taken into account. Until progress is made in the accuracy and reliability of the biomechanical models in representing individual patients, the assessment of muscle length and function on the basis of these models should be approached with great caution.

ORTHOPAEDIC TREATMENT OF MUSCLE

Orthopaedic surgical interventions for muscle problems in CP include primarily lengthening of the muscle-tendon unit. Although tendon lengthening is possible, typically, the aponeurotic lengthening at the musculotendinous junction is preferred, as it is believed to preserve the length ratio between muscle and tendon, thus maximizing strength preservation. It has been shown that muscles in CP are weak and that SEMLS further compromises muscle strength, leading to profound and prolonged weakness (Seniorou et al. 2007). The mechanism through which muscle strength is lost after muscle-tendon lengthening is probably multi-factorial. Increasing the length of the muscle-tendon affects the length-strength ratio of the muscle and alters the optimal length of the unit, where maximum strength can be displayed. The altered sarcomere length reported elsewhere in this chapter is probably also involved. Reduced postoperative mobility, pain inhibition, and surgical scarring may also contribute to the problem. Some muscle groups, e.g. the hamstrings, may take a year to recover their preoperative strength. However, surgical interventions designed to improve the lever-arm of a muscle group (e.g. hip abductors – correction of femoral anteversion) have been shown to improve postoperative strength (Seniorou et al. 2007).

The implication of these findings is that achieving the 'correct' muscle length for optimal muscle function is the desirable result of muscle/tendon lengthening surgical interventions. There are several challenges in achieving this. First, the 'dose' of lengthening is relatively arbitrary and depends primarily on the experience and training of the surgeon. There is no established and widely accepted method to reliably assess and measure the amount of lengthening necessary to optimize the result of surgery. Second, the surgical technique used for lengthening may be important in optimizing muscle length and preserving strength, but the evidence on which technique is more effective is lacking. Minimally invasive techniques have been suggested to minimize muscle trauma and postoperative pain, thus promoting early and fast rehabilitation (Thompson et al. 2010). Early results were encouraging in terms of strength preservation. As the minimally invasive techniques involved a whole range of SEMLS procedures, it is difficult to assess what the net effect of percutaneous muscle lengthening was. A recent study comparing open versus percutaneous lengthening of the hamstrings demonstrated comparable effectiveness (Nazareth et al. 2019). However, Mansoor et al. showed that percutaneous hamstrings lengthening could cause muscle injury, although this may depend on the surgical technique (2017). Another study demonstrated that surgical release at the musculotendinous junction of the hamstrings followed by slow and gradual postoperative lengthening led to optimal recovery with no significant loss of strength (Davids et al. 2019).

Muscle-tendon lengthening has been discussed at length in the orthopaedic literature on the management of children with CP. This is probably because muscle lengthening is the most obvious surgical solution for children with apparently tight muscles. This does not necessarily mean it is the right solution. As discussed above, there are complex issues affecting CP muscle, other than length, that our imprecise surgical lengthening does not address. In addition, the neurological control of muscle, in the presence of spasticity and dystonia, and compromised selective control, usually remains unaltered following surgical muscle lengthening.

Bony surgery has increasingly replaced muscle lengthening as the central focus of SEMLS in recent years. There is a trend towards indirect muscle lengthening through bone shortening during osteotomy surgery to correct sagittal, coronal, or transverse plane deformities (Healy et al. 2011). Complex three-dimensional corrections, such as the supracondylar extension derotation femoral osteotomy, may not always produce predictable results in terms of muscle length alterations. Musculoskeletal modeling may be helpful to calculate the effect of bony correction on muscle length – a recent study elegantly demonstrated the effect of supracondylar femoral osteotomy on hamstrings length (Lenhart et al. 2017). Another important role of bony surgery is the optimization of muscle function through correction of pathological lever arms. This is discussed in Chapter 1 of this book. In the context of SEMLS, muscle-tendon operations are undertaken in combination with bony procedures. Therefore, studying the net effect of each surgical procedure is challenging.

Another surgical technique used in the management of muscle in CP involves transferring tendon attachments, altering the function of the muscle-tendon unit. The aim is to use the transferred muscle activity in order to correct a pathological function. Tibialis anterior or posterior (split) transfer around the foot and rectus femoris or proximal semitendinosus transfer around the knee are the most common examples in the lower limb. As a principle, for a transfer to work effectively, the muscle has to be under adequate voluntary control or to consistently show phasic pathological activity at an appropriate time of the gait cycle to produce the desired effect. The transferred muscle should also have adequate strength to achieve the desired effect, taking into account that the transfer itself leads to some loss of strength, at least temporarily (Piazza et al. 2003). It is possible that the effectiveness of some of these operations is not based on an adequately functioning transferred muscle but on the tenodesis (internal bracing) effect or the de-activation of the muscle's pathological function before the transfer.

Tendon shortening has also been suggested as a surgical method to reduce the length of the muscle-tendon unit in order to optimize strength and function. Shortening of the patellar tendon is routinely used during correction of knee joint contractures (Sossai et al. 2015). Shortening of the tibialis anterior tendon in combination with plantar flexor lengthening has been shown to produce satisfactory and lasting results in correcting equinus gait (Kläusler et al. 2017).

Postoperative rehabilitation is an integral part of the orthopaedic treatment of CP muscle. Although there is some evidence that resistance-based physiotherapy regimes carry advantages (Seniorou et al. 2007), there is little evidence-based practice in the postoperative management of this population (Amirmudin et al. 2019). Research studies that define the optimal physiotherapy regimes for preoperative conditioning and postoperative rehabilitation are clearly necessary.

TREATMENT OUTCOMES

Treatment outcomes are discussed at length in Chapter 3 of this book. Focusing specifically on muscle, the general principle of preserving or improving strength and function and alleviating or preventing pain through treatment would still apply. Achieving these aims would contribute towards a stable and energy-efficient physical function.

Although many outcome measures for the evaluation of clinical results are in use, their application in the research context is largely inconsistent. The consequences of research heterogeneity in outcome measures across studies limits the ability to compare findings among studies. Generic and clinician-administrated outcome measures, such as clinical measurements of joint range of motion, spasticity, muscle strength, and instrumented gait analysis, are employed in most CP orthopaedic literature, leaving the needs and expectations of both patient and caregivers unfulfilled. Such inadequate reporting renders these studies less reliable and further reduces the ability to compare and combine studies through meta-analysis.

The Core Outcome Measures in Effectiveness Trials initiative brings together researchers interested in developing a standardized set of core outcomes in different health-related fields (COMET n.d). A core outcome set is defined as 'an agreed minimum set of outcomes that is recommended to be measured and reported in all clinical trials.' (COMET n.d). A Core Outcome Set is developed through a process that includes literature review, interviews, and surveys of all stakeholders, including patients and families, and a final consensus meeting.

Given the inconsistency, heterogeneity, irrelevance, and reporting bias in outcome domains and measures identified in studies on lower limb surgery for ambulant CP, it is important to develop a core outcome set that specifically addresses the needs of children and young people with CP undergoing lower-limb orthopaedic surgery. A search of the Core Outcome Measures in Effectiveness Trials database and existing literature revealed that a core outcome set development has not been undertaken for the orthopaedic surgical management of lower limb problems in CP. This appears to be an immediate research need in this area, currently pursued at Oxford, where early findings from this process indicate that pain, surgical adverse events, improved balance, and ability to cope with activities of daily living and hobbies are rated highly by stakeholders who do not have a health professional background.

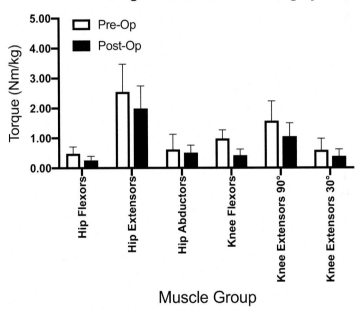

Figure 7.8 Percentage change in strength of lower limb muscles at 1 year following conventional single-stage multi-level surgery and minimally invasive – strength preserving surgery: differences in knee extensors and knee flexors are significant.

FUTURE NEEDS

Feasible and realistic goals for the next 5 years

- Establish a widely agreed core outcome set to be used in the study of lower limb interventions in cerebral palsy (CP). Until this is achieved, there will be no consistency of outcomes in the published literature and no ability to undertake meaningful meta-analysis.

- Plan prospective randomized controlled clinical trials comparing different regimes in the preoperative conditioning and postoperative rehabilitation in single-event multilevel surgery (SEMLS). In the UK there is currently a national study collecting prospective data on all SEMLS patients (CPinBOSS n..d). This should provide sufficient baseline data to allow meaningful comparisons of surgical techniques and rehabilitation techniques in the future.
- Development and expansion of muscle and muscle-tendon length modeling.
- Modeling of the neurological control and strength of muscle is more challenging, and should remain a longer-term aim.

REFERENCES

Amirmudin NA, Lavelle G, Theologis T, Thompson N, Ryan JM (2019) Multilevel surgery for children with cerebral palsy: a meta-analysis. *Pediatrics* **143**: e20183390.

Bar-On L, Molenaers G, Aertbeliën E, et al. (2015) Spasticity and its contribution to hypertonia in cerebral palsy. *Biomed Res Int* **2015**: 317047.

Bodine SC, Roy RR, Meadows DA et al. (1982) Architectural, histochemical, and contractile characteristics of a unique biarticular muscle: the cat semitendinosus. *J Neurophysiol* **48**: 192–201.

Brand, PW, Hollister A. (1993). *Clinical Mechanics of the Hand*. St. Louis, MO: Mosby.

Brown SH, Ward SR, Cook MS, Lieber RL (2011) Architectural analysis of human abdominal wall muscles: implications for mechanical function. *Spine* **36**: 355–362.

Burkholder TJ, Lieber RL (2001) Sarcomere length operating range of muscles during movement. *J Exp Biol* **204**: 1529–1536.

Cerebral Palsy in the British Orthopaedic Surveillance Study – CPinBOSS (n.d) CPinBOSS, viewed in 2020 https://www.ndorms.ox.ac.uk/clinical-trials/current-trials-and-studies/cpinboss-study

Choi JY, Park ES, Park D, Rha DW (2018) Dynamic spasticity determines hamstring length and knee flexion angle during gait in children with spastic cerebral palsy. *Gait Posture* **64**: 255–259.

Cleworth DR, Edman KAP (1972) Changes in sarcomere length during isometric tension development in frog skeletal muscle. *J Physiol* **227**: 1–17.

Core Outcome Measures in Effectiveness Trials – COMET (n.d) COMET, viewed in 2020 http://www.comet-initiative.org/

Dallmeijer AJ, Baker R, Dodd KJ, Taylor NF (2011) Association between isometric muscle strength and gait joint kinetics in adolescents and young adults with cerebral palsy. *Gait Posture* **33**: 326–332.

Dayanidhi S, Lieber RL (2014) Skeletal muscle satellite cells: mediators of muscle growth during development and implications for developmental disorders. *Muscle Nerve* **50**: 723–732.

Davids JR, Cung NQ, Sattler K, Boakes JL, Bagley AM (2019) Quantitative Assessment of Muscle Strength Following "Slow" Surgical Lengthening of the Medial Hamstring Muscles in Children With Cerebral Palsy. *J Pediatr Orthop* **39**: e373–e379.

Dayanidhi S, Dykstra PB, Lyubasyuk V, McKay BR, Chambers HG, Lieber RL (2015) Reduced satellite cell number in situ in muscular contractures from children with cerebral palsy. *J Orthop Res* **33**: 1039–1045.

Domenighetti AA, Mathewson MA, Pichika R et al. (2018) Loss of myogenic potential and fusion capacity of muscle stem cells isolated from contractured muscle in children with cerebral palsy. *Am J Physiol Cell Physiol* **315**: C247–C257.

Edman K (1966) The relation between sarcomere length and active tension in isolated semitendinosus fibres of the frog. *J Physiol* **183**: 407–417.

Enoka R (1994) *Neuromechanical basis of kinesiology*. Champaign: Human Kinetics.

Feige P, Brun CE, Ritso M, Rudnicki MA (2018) Orienting Muscle Stem Cells for Regeneration in Homeostasis, Aging, and Disease. *Cell stem cell* **23**: 653–664.

Fridén J (2005) *Tendon Transfers in Reconstructive Hand Surgery*. Oxford: Taylor and Francis.

Fridén J, Lieber RL (1994) Physiologic consequences of surgical lengthening of extensor carpi radialis brevis muscle-tendon junction for tennis elbow. *J Hand Surg Am* **19**: 269–274.

Fridén J, Lieber RL (2002) Tendon transfer surgery: clinical implications of experimental studies. *Clin Orthop Relat Res* **2002**: S163–S170.

Fridén J, Lieber RL (2003) Spastic muscle cells are shorter and stiffer than normal cells. *Muscle Nerve* **27**: 157–164.

Gage JR (2007) *The Treatment of Gait Problems in Cerebral Palsy.* Cambridge: Mac Keith Press.

Gans C, Gaunt AS (1991) Muscle architecture in relation to function. *J Biomech* **24S1**: 53–65.

Geister TL, Quintanar-Solares M, Martin M, Aufhammer S, Asmus F (2014) Qualitative development of the 'Questionnaire on Pain caused by Spasticity (QPS),' a pediatric patient-reported outcome for spasticity-related pain in cerebral palsy. *Qual Life Res* **23**: 887–896.

Gillies AM, Lieber RL (2011) Structure and function of the skeletal muscle extracellular matrix. *Muscle Nerve* **44**: 318–331.

Gillies AR, Chapman MA, Bushong EA, Deerinck TJ, Ellisman MH, Lieber RL (2017) High resolution three-dimensional reconstruction of fibrotic skeletal muscle extracellular matrix. *J Physiol* **595**: 1159–1171.

Gokhin DS, Bang ML, Zhang J, Chen J, Lieber RL (2009) Reduced thin filament length in nebulin-knockout skeletal muscle alters isometric contractile properties. *Am J Physiol Cell Physiol* **296**: C1123–C1132.

Gordon AM, Huxley AF, Julian FJ (1966) The variation in isometric tension with sarcomere length in vertebrate muscle fibres. *J Physiol* **184**: 170–192.

Healy MT, Schwartz MH, Stout JL, Gage JR, Novacheck TF (2011) Is simultaneous hamstring lengthening necessary when performing distal femoral extension osteotomy and patellar tendon advancement? *Gait Posture* **33**: 1–5.

Kläusler M, Speth BM, Brunner R, Tirosh O, Camathias C, Rutz E (2017) Long-term follow-up after tibialis anterior tendon shortening in combination with Achilles tendon lengthening in spastic equinus in cerebral palsy. *Gait Posture* **58**: 457–462.

Lenhart RL, Smith CR, Schwartz MH, Novacheck TF, Thelen DG (2017) The effect of distal femoral extension osteotomy on muscle lengths after surgery. *J Child Orthop* **11**: 472–478.

Leung AF (1982) Calculation of the laser diffraction intensity of striated muscle by numerical methods. *Comput Programs Biomed* **15**: 169–174.

Lieber RL (2010) *Skeletal muscle structure and function and plasticity.* Baltimore: Lippincott, Williams & Wilkins.

Lieber RL, Fazeli BM, Botte MJ (1990) Architecture of selected wrist flexor and extensor muscles. *J Hand Surg* **15A**: 244–250.

Lieber RL, Fridén J (1997) Intraoperative measurement and biomechanical modeling of the flexor carpi ulnaris-to-extensor carpi radialis longus tendon transfer. *J Biomech Eng* **119**: 386–391.

Lieber RL, Fridén J (2000) Functional and clinical significance of skeletal muscle architecture. *Muscle Nerve* **23**: 1647–1666.

Lieber RL, Fridén J (2002) Spasticity causes a fundamental rearrangement of muscle-joint interaction. *Muscle & Nerve* **25**: 265–270.

Lieber RL, Jacobson MD, Fazeli BM, Abrams RA, Botte MJ (1992) Architecture of selected muscles of the arm and forearm: anatomy and implications for tendon transfer. *J Hand Surg* **17A**: 787–798.

Lieber RL, Loren GJ, Fridén J (1994) In vivo measurement of human wrist extensor muscle sarcomere length changes. *J Neurophysiol* **71**: 874–881.

Lieber RL, Murray W, Clark DL, Hentz VR, Fridén J (2005) Biomechanical properties of the brachioradialis muscle: implications for surgical tendon transfer. *J Hand Surg* **30**: 273–282.

Lieber RL, Pontén E, Burkholder TJ, Fridén J (1996) Sarcomere length changes after flexor carpi ulnaris-to-extensor digitorum communis tendon transfer. *J Hand Surg* **21A**: 612–618.

Lieber RL, Runesson E, Einarsson F, Friden J (2003) Inferior mechanical properties of spastic muscle bundles due to hypertrophic but compromised extracellular matrix material. *Muscle Nerve* **28**: 464–471.

Lieber RL, Yeh Y, Baskin RJ (1984) Sarcomere length determination using laser diffraction. Effect of beam and fiber diameter. *Biophys J* **45**: 1007–1016.

Ljung B-O, Lieber RL, Fridén J (1999) Wrist extensor muscle pathology in in lateral epicondylitis. *Journal of Hand Surgery* **24:** 177–183.

Ljung B-O, Fridén J, Lieber RL (1999) Sarcomere length varies with wrist ulnar deviation but not forearm pronation in the extensor carpi radialis brevis muscle. *J Biomech* **32**: 199–202.

Mansour T, Derienne J, Daher M, Sarraf D, Zoghbi Y, Ghanem I (2017) Is percutaneous medial hamstring lengthening as anatomically effective and safe as the open procedure? *J Child Orthop* **11**: 15–19.

Mathewson MA, Ward SR, Chambers HG, Lieber RL (2015) High resolution muscle measurements provide insights into equinus contractures in patients with cerebral palsy. *J Orthop Res* **33**: 33–39.

Meseguer-Henarejos AB, Sánchez-Meca J, López-Pina JA, Carles-Hernández R (2018) Inter- and intra-rater reliability of the Modified Ashworth Scale: a systematic review and meta-analysis. *Eur J Phys Rehabil Med* **54**: 576–590.

Murray WM, Buchanan TS, Delp SL (2000) The isometric functional capacity of muscles that cross the elbow. *J Biomech* **33**: 943–952.

Nazareth A, Rethlefsen S, Sousa TC, Mueske NM, Wren TAL, Kay RM (2019) Percutaneous Hamstring Lengthening Surgery is as Effective as Open Lengthening in Children With Cerebral Palsy. *J Pedia Orthop* **39**: 366–371.

Piazza SJ, Adamson RL, Moran MF, Sanders JO, Sharkey NA (2003) Effects of tensioning errors in split transfers of tibialis anterior and posterior tendons. *Bone Joint Surg Am* **85**: 858–865.

Powell PL, Roy RR, Kanim P, Bello M, Edgerton VR (1984) Predictability of skeletal muscle tension from architectural determinations in guinea pig hindlimbs. *J Appl Physiol* **57**: 1715–1721.

Rang M, Wenger D (1993) *The Art and Practice of Children's Orthopaedics*. Philadelphia: Lippincott, Williams and Wilkins.

Rha DW, Cahill-Rowley K, Young J et al. (2016) Biomechanical and Clinical Correlates of Stance-Phase Knee Flexion in Persons With Spastic Cerebral Palsy. *PM R* **8**: 11–18.

Rüdel R, Zite FF (1980) Efficiency of light diffraction by cross-striated muscle fibers under stretch and during isometric contraction. *Biophys J* **30**: 507–516.

Salami F, Wagner J, van Drongelen S, et al. (2018) Mid-term development of hamstring tendon length and velocity after distal femoral extension osteotomy in children with bilateral cerebral palsy: a retrospective cohort study. *Dev Med Child Neurol* **60**: 833–838.

Schwartz MH, Rozumalski A, Steele KM (2016) Dynamic motor control is associated with treatment outcomes for children with cerebral palsy. *Dev Med Child Neurol* **58**: 1139–1145.

Seniorou M, Thompson N, Harrington M, Theologis T (2007) Recovery of muscle strength following multi-level orthopaedic surgery in diplegic cerebral palsy. *Gait Posture* **26**: 475–481.

Smith LR, Chambers HG, Lieber RL (2013) Reduced satellite cell population may lead to contractures in children with cerebral palsy. *Dev Med Child Neurol* **55**: 264–270.

Smith LR, Chambers HG, Subramaniam S, Lieber RL (2012) Transcriptional abnormalities of hamstring muscle contractures in children with cerebral palsy. *PloS one* **7**: e40686.

Smith LR, Lee KS, Ward SR, Chambers HG, Lieber RL (2011) Hamstring contractures in children with spastic cerebral palsy result from a stiffer extracellular matrix and increased in vivo sarcomere length. *J Physiol* **589**: 2625–2639.

Smith LR, Pichika R, Meza RC et al. (2019) Contribution of extracellular matrix components to the stiffness of skeletal muscle contractures in patients with cerebral palsy. *Connect Tissue Res* **2019**: 1–12.

Sossai R, Vavken P, Brunner R, Camathias C, Graham HK, Rutz E (2015) Patellar tendon shortening for flexed knee gait in spastic diplegia. *Gait Posture* **41**: 658–665.

Tabary JC, Tabary C, Tardieu C, Tardieu G, Goldspink G (1972) Physiological and structural changes in the cat's soleus muscle due to immobilization at different lengths by plaster casts. *J Physiol* **224**: 231–244.

Takahashi M, Ward S, Lieber RL (2007) Intraoperative single-site sarcomere length measurement accurately reflects whole muscle sarcomere length. *J Hand Surg* **32**: 612–617.

Takahashi M, Ward SR, Friden J, Lieber RL (2012) Muscle excursion does not correlate with increased serial sarcomere number after muscle adaptation to stretched tendon transfer. *J Orthop Res* **30**: 1774–1780.

Thompson N, Stebbins J, Seniorou M, Newham D (2011) Muscle strength and walking ability in diplegic cerebral palsy: implications for assessment and management. *Gait Posture* **33**: 321–325.

Thompson N, Stebbins J, Seniorou M, Wainwright AM, Newham DJ, Theologis TN (2010) The use of minimally invasive techniques in multi-level surgery for children with cerebral palsy: preliminary results. *J Bone Joint Surg Br* **92**: 1442–1448.

Ward SR, Eng CM, Smallwood LH, Lieber RL (2009) Are current measurements of lower extremity muscle architecture accurate? *Clin Orthop Relat Res* **467**: 1074–1082.

Ward SR, Kim CW, Eng CM et al. (2009) Architectural analysis and intraoperative measurements demonstrate the unique design of the multifidus muscle for lumbar spine stability. *J Bone Joint Surg Am* **91**: 176–185.

Williams PE, Goldspink G (1971) Longitudinal growth of striated muscle fibres. *J Cell Sci* **9**: 751–767.

Wickiewicz TL, Roy RR, Powell PL, Edgerton VR (1983) Muscle architecture of the human lower limb. *Clin Orthop Rel Res* **179**: 275–283.

Williams P, Goldspink G (1973) The effect of immobilization on the longitudinal growth of striated muscle fibers. *J Anat* **116**: 45–55.

Winters TM, Takahashi M, Lieber RL, Ward SR (2011) Whole muscle length-tension relationships are accurately modeled as scaled sarcomeres in rabbit hindlimb muscles. *J Biomech* **44**: 109–115.

Pathomorphology of Skeletal Muscle in Cerebral Palsy
Current State and New Directions

Jason J Howard, H Kerr Graham, and Adam P Shortland

KEY POINTS

- Understanding the pathophysiology of skeletal muscle in cerebral palsy (CP) is paramount to developing and applying interventions that reduce contracture while preserving strength.
- The 'traditional view' whereby spastic/dynamic muscle contractures lead to fixed contractures and bony deformities, is likely incorrect and needs reconsideration in light of recent studies.
- Sarcomeres, the basic contractile unit of skeletal muscle, are long and may contribute to the muscle weakness seen in children with CP.
- Fixed muscle contractures are related to increases in connective tissue, possibly an adaptive mechanism in the face of increased in vivo muscle tension.
- Titin, a spring-like molecule that supports the sarcomere at its ends, is negatively affected in CP, resulting in highly elastic myofibrils and possibly accounting for decreases in eccentric muscle force.
- DNA methylation is abnormal in CP and may be responsible for abnormalities in muscle growth and function.
- Botulinum neurotoxin A (BoNT-A) causes muscle atrophy and upregulation of fibrofatty connective tissue in animal models, consistent with the lack of functional improvement seen in recent human studies.
- Further study is needed to understand the effect of muscle lengthening surgery on function, but changes in fascicle length and pennation angles have been observed.

Musculoskeletal manifestations in spastic cerebral palsy (CP) have been attributed to cortical and subcortical injuries in the developing brain. Abnormalities of skeletal muscle function in CP have traditionally been considered a consequence of sustained activation of dominant muscle groups forcing joints into abnormal postures, with adaptive shortening of the muscle-tendon-unit and the development of fixed contractures (Graham et al. 2016). Many believe that this active shortening results, ultimately, in fixed contracture as the muscle adapts to a new operating point of activation (Hof 2001; Graham and Selber 2003). In this simple, linear sequence, bony deformity occurs secondary to an imbalance of muscle forces; resulting in abnormal torsional and bending stresses that induce abnormal bone growth (Rang 1990; Lynn et al. 2009). This model has influenced orthopedic management in spastic CP over the last 50 years, with practitioners seeking to reduce muscle activation through pharmaceutical or surgical intervention(s). In doing so, the underlying belief was that these interventions would delay the development of deformity, restore joint range of motion through muscle lengthening, and subsequently modify bone geometry to improve alignment.

Recent advances in our understanding of neurodevelopment, muscle growth and composition, and the bone-muscle unit, have called this 'traditional view' of deformity development into question. This viewpoint has been amplified by the disappointing outcomes of long-term studies of spasticity reduction interventions. In this chapter, we will review these research studies and discuss how they may influence the application of orthopedic and spasticity management going forward.

THE ROLE OF SPASTICITY IN MUSCLE CONTRACTURE: CHALLENGING THE TRADITIONAL VIEW

The 'traditional view', illustrated by Rang's three stages of CP, may not represent the full story (Fig. 8.1, [Rang 1990]). At the hip, for example, though prolonged spastic/dynamic adductor and flexor contractures have been implicated as a primary driver of hip displacement (i.e. subluxation, dislocation), focal spasticity management by botulinum neurotoxin A (BoNT-A) injections of these muscles has neither resulted in its prevention nor resolution, even when combined with abduction bracing (Graham et al. 2008; Willoughby et al. 2012). In addition, there is no evidence that global spasticity management – either by intrathecal baclofen or dorsal rhizotomy – reduces the development of muscle contractures, frequency of hip displacement, or the need for orthopedic surgery in CP (Miller et al. 2017; Tedroff et al. 2019).

The influence of motor type is also an issue to consider. Although the spastic motor type is most prevalent in CP, representing 86% of children in a population-based cohort from Melbourne, a small number are hypotonic, typically without static contracture (Howard et al. 2005). In this same cohort of patients, the overall incidence of hip displacement was 35% and was found to be unrelated to motor type (Soo et al. 2006). Indeed, hip displacement was present in 44% of children with hypotonia – typified by lateral physeal tilt, coxa valga, and acetabular dysplasia – despite having neither spasticity nor adductor contractures. Therefore, it has been suggested that the true cause of hip displacement may be secondary to abductor weakness, with the physis realigning itself to tilt more laterally according to the resultant force on the hip joint (Howard et al. 2019). The subsequent increase in the femoral neck-shaft angle imparts lateral pressure at the acetabular margin, resulting in a progressive dysplasia (Tachdjian and Minear 1956; Phelps 1959; Robin et al. 2008; Gose et al. 2010; Lee et al. 2010; Graham et al. 2016). Corroborating this theory, similar patterns of femoral and acetabular deformity are typical for other primarily hypotonic neuromuscular disorders. For example, in spinal muscular atrophy, lateral physeal tilt and coxa valga of the proximal femur have been suggested to result from an absence or delay in weight-bearing, in addition to abductor insufficiency (Larson and Snyder 2019). Given these findings, it would seem that a more unifying mechanism lies in the negative features of CP rather than the positive (Fig. 8.2).

In ambulatory CP, the reduction of spasticity by injection of BoNT-A has also had little effect on the prevention of static contracture or the need for subsequent orthopedic surgery. Injection of BoNT-A is the most common medical intervention in children with CP (Graham 2016). There is good evidence that injection of BoNT-A can delay the need for surgery in ankle equinus, although other interventions such as serial casting, physiotherapy, and the use of orthoses may also achieve the same goal. There is no evidence that injections of BoNT-A can prevent the development of fixed contractures or bony torsional deformities and the need for orthopedic surgery (Koman et al. 1993; Molenears et al. 2006).

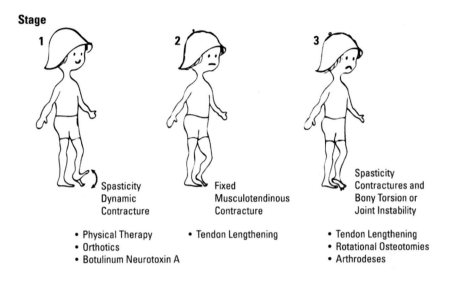

Stage

1
Spasticity
Dynamic
Contracture

2
Fixed
Musculotendinous
Contracture

3
Spasticity
Contractures and
Bony Torsion or
Joint Instability

- Physical Therapy
- Orthotics
- Botulinum Neurotoxin A

- Tendon Lengthening

- Tendon Lengthening
- Rotational Osteotomies
- Arthrodeses

Figure 8.1 Rang's three stages of cerebral palsy, illustrating the 'traditional view' with (1) spastic/dynamic muscle contractures (without shortening) leading to (2) fixed/static muscle contractures (with shortening). (3) Abnormal muscle forces secondary to spasticity and muscle shortening then lead to bony deformations, including abnormal torsion and coronal deviations such as increased femoral anteversion and coxa valga. This intuitive view has supported a pervasive rationale for the treatment of spasticity: to prevent contractures and bony deformation, and thus, orthopedic surgery. Given the results of recent prospective studies and systematic reviews which refute the effect of spasticity management on muscle and bone, this view is being challenged. Used with permission © Bill Reid / Kerr Graham, RCH Melbourne.

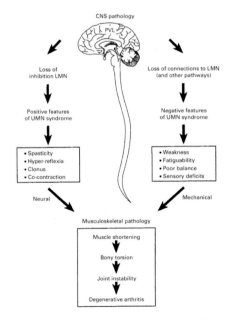

Figure 8.2 Positive and negative features of the cerebral palsy upper motor neuron syndrome. Negative features such as weakness (graphic right side) are likely more important in the development of bony deformities (e.g. abductor weakness as a cause of coxa valga of the proximal femur) rather than positive features such as spasticity. Muscle stiffness, recently found to be secondary to an upregulation of the collagen-based extracellular matrix, may develop in parallel with, rather than secondary to, spasticity. Used with permission, © Kerr Graham, RCH Melbourne.

The original thinking behind the introduction of BoNT-A for CP was based on the view that the treatment of dynamic contractures would affect the onset of fixed contracture and thus bony deformity (Cosgrove and Graham 1994). However, there is little evidence to support this intuitive view. In a study by Alhusseini and colleagues, although BoNT-A injections into the calf muscle reliably decreased muscle tone (the 'R1' or spastic catch by the Modified Tardieu Scale [Yam et al. 2006]), the authors reported no improvements in passive range of motion nor stiffness (i.e. static contracture [Alhusaini et al. 2011]). In addition, this reduction in muscle tone came at the expense of muscle torque. Another study from Sweden investigating the long-term effects of BoNT-A in CP found prolonged reduction of tone but no evidence of static contracture prevention over 3 years post-injection (Tedroff et al. 2009).

The use of selective dorsal rhizotomy (SDR) has become popular for spasticity reduction using a more global approach, particularly for ambulatory CP. This technique involves the selective sectioning of afferent nerve fibers where they enter the dorsal nerve root of the spinal cord, decreasing efferent excitation. In one study with over 10 years follow-up post-SDR, spasticity was reliably reduced, but functional gains were not realized over and above what would be expected from a child without SDR, following their Gross Motor Function Measure (GMFM-66) curve in accordance with their Gross Motor Function Classification System level (Tedroff et al. 2011). Despite an initial increase in range of motion in lower extremity joints, by 10 years post-SDR, static contractures at the hip and knee developed in spite of the spasticity reduction. Adding to this, 84% of children in this study underwent orthopedic surgery (20% by 3 years post-SDR). With the exception of further deterioration in gross motor function, a follow-up report on this same cohort at 17 years post-SDR gave largely the same results (Tedroff et al. 2015). These findings were corroborated in a systematic review by Novak and colleagues (2013). In addition to the lack of efficacy in preventing static contractures, it has also been conceded that SDR has little effect on the development of bony deformities and 'lever arm dysfunction' in ambulatory CP (Wang et al. 2018). As such, in addition to muscle lengthening procedures, the need for derotational osteotomies of the femur and tibia in single-event multilevel surgery for gait correction will likely still be required. This is not to say that SDR has no role in CP. Its success in permanently reducing spasticity likely has other benefits relating to the relief of painful spasms and improvements in health-related quality of life measures. Its role in static contracture prevention, however, needs reconsideration.

Regarding the development of bony deformity in CP, there is good evidence from large population-based studies that medial femoral torsion stems from a persistent increase in femoral neck anteversion and not as a result of spasticity-mediated deforming forces under the influence of growth (Robin et al. 2008). In addition, there is evidence that external tibial torsion is acquired during growth as a result of disordered gait biomechanics and, once again, is not the result of spasticity (Graham 2014; Graham et al. 2016).

Another more global approach to spasticity management involves the use of intrathecal baclofen. Baclofen is a gamma-aminobutyric acid agonist which impedes the action of excitatory neurotransmitters in the spinal cord, delivered by an implanted pump. Despite some evidence regarding its efficacy for reducing spasticity and improving quality of life, there is a paucity of well-designed studies that evaluate its role in the prevention of contractures or bony deformity (Albright et al. 1991; Hasnat and Rice 2015).

In summary, it would seem that spasticity reduction, regardless of how it is achieved, does little to prevent muscle shortening in CP and does not reliably reduce the need for orthopedic surgery.

SARCOMERE DYSFUNCTION IN CP: A CAUSE OF MUSCLE WEAKNESS

Effective muscle function is dependent on the ability to generate force, subsequently applied to skeletal levers to propel body movement and ambulation. Muscles are arranged hierarchically into contractile and non-contractile elements to generate force and as a structural scaffold, respectively (Fig. 8.3).

The basic unit of muscle contraction is the sarcomere, arranged in series as myofibrils, which are bundled into muscle fibers (Fig 8.3a). Sarcomeres are comprised of both actin (thin) and myosin (thick) myofilaments that slide over each other during muscle contraction according to the sliding filament theory (Huxley and Niedergerke 1954) (Fig. 8.4). The force-generating ability of each sarcomere is dependent on its length, approximately 2.5µm in typically developing children, but excessively long in CP averaging approximately 3.5μm (Smith et al. 2011; Leonard et al. 2019) (Fig. 8.3b). At these longer lengths, their force-generating capacity is dramatically reduced according to the Gordon-Huxley-Julian sarcomere force-length relation (Gordon et al. 1966). Accordingly, these overly long sarcomeres are very likely responsible for the muscle weakness seen as a primary negative feature in CP.

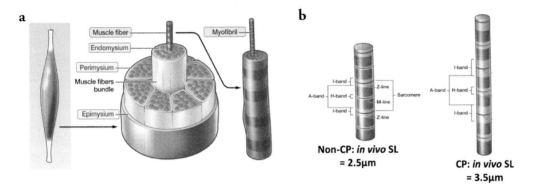

a

b

Non-CP: *in vivo* SL = 2.5µm

CP: *in vivo* SL = 3.5µm

Figure 8.3 (a) Basic muscle hierarchy demonstrating contractile (pink) and non-contractile (orange) elements. (b) Comparison of sarcomere lengths for myofibrils in cerebral palsy (CP) and typically developing children. At their typically long in vivo sarcomere lengths, CP muscle can be expected to generate less force secondary to suboptimal actin and myosin overlap, as compared to typically developing children. Used with permission © Bill Reid / Kerr Graham, RCH Melbourne.

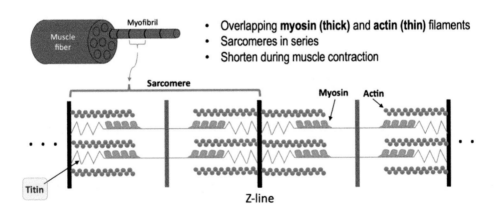

- Overlapping **myosin (thick)** and **actin (thin)** filaments
- Sarcomeres in series
- Shorten during muscle contraction

Figure 8.4 Sarcomeres are comprised of overlapping myosin and actin myofilaments that slide over one another to produce a contractile force according to the sliding filament theory. Sarcomeres are stabilized at their ends by a large protein named titin: a spring-like molecule that mainly tethers the thick filaments to the Z-line, and is primarily responsible for myofibril stiffness. Graphic by Jason J Howard.

The mismatch of resting (i.e. in vivo) and optimal sarcomere lengths in CP muscle may have other important consequences. When resting length and optimal active length are similar, muscles may develop forces quickly from a resting state once activated. The slow rate of development of force in muscle in spastic CP may well be related to the minimal overlap of actin and myosin in the sarcomere at rest. To obtain an optimal functional position, elongated sarcomeres must shorten, reducing muscle length, and forcing the joint into an abnormal position. Sarcomere elongation, then, would explain phenomena that we often consider to be 'neurological' in origin, such as dynamic equinus, dynamic hamstring shortness (crouch gait), and increased muscle coactivation. Deficits in muscle growth, composition, and energetics become more apparent with age, and it may be that these shortened optimal active lengths cannot be maintained during normal functional activities such as walking (Kalsi et al. 2016).

The mechanisms underlying this phenomenon of sarcomere elongation are unclear. In a study investigating myofibrillar properties in CP adductor muscles, it was found that in vivo sarcomere lengths for myofibrils were under significantly increased tension compared to typically developing controls (Leonard et al. 2019). Perhaps this increased tension has stretched the sarcomeres to their limit, accounting for their increased length and subsequent muscle weakness. Alternatively, the increase in sarcomere length under stress could be an adaptive mechanism.

Sarcomeres are stabilized at their ends by a large protein named titin. Titin is a spring-like molecule that mainly tethers the thick filaments to the Z-line, and is primarily responsible for myofibril stiffness, the sarcomere otherwise being devoid of other structural elements (Fig. 8.4) (Herzog 2014). The molecule is comprised of an immunoglobulin domain that unfolds as it is stretched. Once sarcomeres are stretched beyond their optimal actin-myosin overlap (as in the case of overstretched sarcomeres in CP), titin alone has been shown to be responsible for the generation of passive force production (i.e. stiffness) in the myofibril (Herzog 2017). Paradoxically, in a study investigating the causes of CP muscle stiffness, Leonard and colleagues found CP hip adductor longus myofibrils to be 40% more elastic than typically developing comparisons with developmental hip dysplasia (Leonard et al. 2019). This increased elasticity was accompanied by a 45% decrease in overall titin amount. This unexpected finding implied an adaptive – perhaps protective – mechanism at work, likely related to changes in the titin isoform and amount that renders the molecule more passively elastic.

In addition to its passive mechanics, titin has been shown to modulate active force generation as well (Labeit et al. 2003), a feature that may have implications for CP muscle. When titin is activated through calcium-binding and phosphorylation at specific titin-binding sites, the amount of myofibrillar force generation has been shown to increase by 3 to 4 times its passive force. This feature has been theorized to explain the increased force enhancement seen in skeletal muscle during eccentric contraction and accounts for the energy efficiency of this action as titin-binding has almost zero cost (Herzog 2017). Since eccentrically contracting muscles, such as the soleus, are essential for energy-efficient ambulation in CP, modulation of titin – pharmacological or otherwise – could provide a means to increase active muscle force generation and thus prevent or treat pathological gait deviations (e.g. crouch).

Investigations into the role of titin in CP muscle, thus far, have been rather rudimentary, focusing on changes in size of this massive molecule rather than its structure and active function. From research investigating the role of titin in CP hip adductor muscles in children with non-ambulatory CP, though the mean size of titin was unchanged, the total amount of titin was decreased in CP versus controls (Leonard et al. 2019) As discussed above, these changes render titin – and hence the myofibril – highly compliant, possibly as an adaptive response to prevent damage from a muscle under substantial tension. In a further investigation of this patient sample, a positive correlation between titin molecular weight and hip displacement (according to migration percentage) was identified (Larkin-Kaiser et al. 2019). These two studies suggest that titin has a role in CP muscle that is related to disease severity, but what causes this is currently unclear. One could theorize that the insult responsible for the development of CP could result in proportional abnormalities in TTN expression – the gene encoding titin – associated with pathological changes in myofibril elasticity and force generation. As discussed in the following section, changes in DNA methylation in response to stress (e.g. an insult to the developing brain) could be responsible for these pathological mechanisms. Supporting this theory, TTN gene hypermethylation has been identified previously in response to exercise stress (Gim et al. 2015). This area of research needs further attention as the important function of titin in normal muscle, both actively and passively, infers that the molecule has a very important role in myofibrillar force generation and thus strength.

Future treatments that both improve actin and myosin overlap and restore the normal elasticity of titin within the sarcomere could provide the means to decrease muscle weakness in CP and subsequently improve function.

IMPAIRED MUSCLE GROWTH IN CP: THE POTENTIAL ROLE OF SATELLITE CELLS

It is well established that CP muscle is not only shortened but also has significant reduction in cross-sectional area, features seen as early as 15 months of age (Gough and Shortland 2012; Noble et al. 2014; Herskind et al. 2016). In addition to mechanically disadvantaged sarcomeres, the reduced cross-sectional area results in decreased muscle strength in CP. CP muscle growth is also known to be impaired, likely tied to a decrease in sarcomerogenesis coupled with a mismatch in bone growth (Gough and Shortland 2012; Pingel et al. 2017). What causes this decrease in muscle growth is not well understood.

One area of recent interest is the role of satellite cells in CP muscle. These stem cells, found sandwiched between the sarcolemma and basal lamina, are responsible for muscle repair and regeneration through the formation of myotubes, which eventually fuse to form myofibers (Yin et al. 2013). These satellite cells have been reliably identified and characterized through the detection of an affiliated molecular marker, the Pax7 transcription factor (Dayanidhi and Lieber 2014). Reduced satellite cell populations of up to 60% have been found in CP as compared to typically developing comparisons, and it has been suggested that this decrease impacts muscle growth and thus strength and excursion (Smith et al. 2013).

In pilot studies, Akins' muscle research group has shown that abnormalities in the expression of Pax7 increase with Gross Motor Function Classification System level, implying a relationship between satellite cell dysfunction and disease severity (Lee et al. 2019). This same research group has identified differences in DNA methylation of CP muscle as compared to typically developing comparisons (Robinson et al. 2019). In epigenetics, DNA methylation is known to be a signalling tool, often indicating that genes are locked in an 'off' position. Sustained abnormalities of DNA methylation within tissue-specific genes, and even genome-wide, have been identified in response to stress, trauma, and disease (Hartley et al. 2013; Houtepen et al. 2016; Sharples et al. 2016; Seaborne et al. 2018). The authors surmised that these epigenetic abnormalities may impair satellite cell function, and thus CP muscle growth.

Crowgey and colleagues have applied machine learning techniques to detect abnormalities in DNA methylation from peripheral blood samples and have reliably identified children with spastic CP from typically developing comparisons (Crowgey et al. 2018) (Fig. 8.5). Demethylating agents are currently available and need further study as a possible treatment to potentially help improve satellite cell function in CP and thus muscle growth. Screening for CP by a simple blood test at an early stage, followed by subsequent treatment of muscle with selective demethylating agents, may allow for more normal muscle growth and sarcomerogenesis (Robert Akins, personal communication, December 2019). If successful, the resulting improvement in the ratio of muscle to bone growth may also serve to prevent contractures. Clearly, this is an advanced concept that needs further exploration.

IF NOT SPASTICITY, WHAT CAUSES MUSCLE STIFFNESS IN CP?

As discussed in the preceding section, *The Role of Spasticity in Muscle Contracture*, the traditional view that spasticity invariably leads to fixed muscle contractures needs reconsideration. But if spasticity is not the culprit, then what is the cause of true muscle stiffness in CP? There is emerging data that suggests one of the main reasons for muscle stiffness lies in the connective tissue scaffold that supports the overall muscle structure.

Non-contractile elements make up a substantial portion of whole muscle, concentrated in the extra-cellular matrix (ECM), which is primarily comprised of Type I collagen (Gilles and Lieber 2011). Surrounding and supporting the contractile muscle fibers, fiber bundles, and the muscle as a whole, the ECM has its own hierarchy, including the endomysium, perimysium, and epimysium (Fig. 8.3). In normal muscle, this highly organized network of collagen cables and perimysial interconnections provide passive structural support and may also have a role in signalling. Pingel and colleagues discussed a potential role for mechanosensitive fibroblasts, which under the adverse mechanical environment applied to CP muscle, may cause a disruption in normal muscle homeostasis (Pingel et al. 2017a). In the previous section, we discussed that CP muscle is under significantly increased tension as compared to muscle in typically developing children (Leonard et al. 2019). It is possible that this increased muscle tension impacts this homeostasis, inducing upregulation of collagen within the ECM and a corresponding increase in passive muscle stiffness. Supporting this theory, biomechanical work has found that passive muscle stiffness increases in proportion to the amount of ECM-based collagen and that this network bears a substantial

a

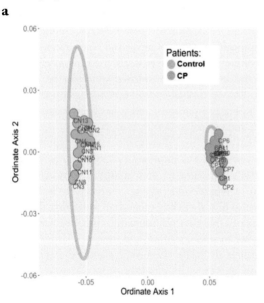

b

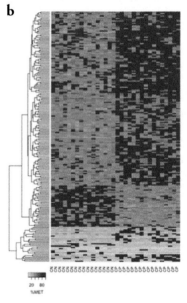

Figure 8.5 (a) Abnormalities in DNA methylation for children with spastic cerebral palsy (CP) versus typically developing comparisons. Cluster analysis of CP versus controls showing distinct differences in DNA methylation. (b) Heatmap clustering of DNA methylation from CP and typically developing comparisons. Yellow = hypomethylated, Blue = hypermethylated (Crowgey et al. 2018). Similar results were preliminarily reported for DNA methylation of skeletal muscle (Robinson et al. 2019). Reprinted from Crowgey et al. 2018 with permission from BioMed Central under the terms of the Creative Commons Attribution 4.0 International License http://creativecommons.org/licenses/by/4.0/.

portion of the total mechanical load on the muscle belly (Alnaqeeb et al. 1984; Gilles and Lieber 2011). Indeed, a growing body of recent evidence suggests that the increased passive stiffness encountered in CP muscle is proportional to increases in ECM-based collagen concentration as compared to typically developing comparisons (Booth et al. 2001; de Bruin et al. 2011; Smith et al. 2011).

An alternative explanation for increased connective tissue content is a lack of myofibrillar development in early life. Herskind and colleagues have shown reduced muscle growth in young children with CP between 6 and 18 months of age (Herskind et al. 2016). In young animal muscle, the myofibrillar proteins to connective tissue content is low. Sustained activation is required for myofibrillar development and connective tissue organisation. It is thought that the development of sustained muscle activation is a consequence of the lowering of alpha motor neuron activation thresholds by the action of a functional corticospinal tract (Clowry 2005). In spastic CP, where the corticospinal tract is damaged, central nervous system development may be delayed, combined with reduced facilitation of alpha motor neurons, decreased and unsustained efferent output to muscles, and resulting in compromised muscle development. With a persistent and unfavourable ratio of myofibrillar to connective tissue, connective tissue structures may be subject to a greater proportion of external load, resulting in increased fibroblast activity.

In response to these findings, it has been hypothesized that the use of a collagenase could (at appropriate dosing) break down the excess collagen in CP muscle ECM to a point which maintains muscle integrity while decreasing stiffness (Howard et al. 2019). This approach has had success for disorders with more densely packed collagen cords – including Dupuytren contracture, Peyronie disease, and uterine fibroids – utilizing collagenase clostridium histolyticum, an enzyme that is highly selective for Type I and Type III collagen that also allows for the preservation of Type IV collagen found in nerves, arteries, and veins (Hurst et al. 2009; Brunengarger et al. 2014; Levine et al. 2014). In view of the complex system likely involved in the maintenance of normal muscle homeostasis, it is recognized that this approach may be overly simplistic, though perhaps no more than what is offered by current treatment modalities. One benefit of a collagen-based approach lies in the preservation of contractile elements for a disorder typified not only by spasticity but, more importantly, by weakness (Multani et al. 2019).

BOTULINUM NEUROTOXIN A: IS THE PRICE OF SPASTICITY MANAGEMENT TOO HIGH?

The use of BoNT-A for the treatment of spasticity in CP was introduced more than 25 years ago, with early basic science work by Cosgrove and Graham, and the first clinical trial by Koman and colleagues in the early 1990s (Cosgrove and Graham 1992; Koman et al. 1993). Until recently, most studies supporting the use of BoNT-A had relatively short follow-up, a situation which led some to call for restraint until more was known about the effects of BoNT-A over the longer term (Gough et al. 2005). Although reductions in hyperreflexia secondary to spasticity were all but guaranteed, there was little evidence to support its role in functional improvement. Indeed, as higher-level evidence with longer-term follow-ups recently became available, systematic reviews have questioned the efficacy of BoNT-A with respect to improvements in function and gait, and expressed concern that there was some evidence for harm (Huntley and Bradley 2017; Multani et al. 2019). In fact, a recent Cochrane review reported that, for studies of at least moderate quality with moderate effect or higher at greater than 6 months post-injection, BoNT-A was not found to be superior to placebo for improvement in gross motor function, range of motion, or even spasticity (Blumetti et al. 2019).

Research groups from Canada, the United States, and Denmark have added animal work to the picture. In a trio of animal studies from Calgary, injections of BoNT-A into lower extremity muscles induced significant reductions in contractile material, which was replaced by increased non-contractile tissue, including fibrosis and fatty infiltration (Fortuna et al. 2011; Fortuna et al. 2013). These findings were still present more than 6 months post-injection and were associated with significant decreases in muscle strength (Fortuna et al. 2015).

Pingel and colleagues confirmed the reduction in muscle mass post-injection in a rat model (by 45%) with concomitant increases in connective tissue and fat (Pingel et al. 2017b). In the previous year, this same research group reported significant decreases in muscle force and increased passive stiffness, in addition to severe muscle atrophy (Pingel et al. 2016). Similar findings were found by Minamoto and colleagues in their rat model (Minamoto et al. 2015).

Despite the increasing number of animal studies reporting the deleterious effects of BoNT-A, there are currently no human histological studies available for review. Despite this, the evidence for muscle atrophy post-BoNT-A injection from human imaging studies is compelling (Schless et al. 2018; Multani et al. 2019). Human muscle tissue studies comparing children with CP to typically developing controls are urgently needed to complete the picture.

Given the preceding discussion regarding the lack of definitive improvement in gross motor function after BoNT-A, coupled with issues relating to the efficacy of spasticity management in CP, a logical question would be: is reduction in spasticity worth the cost? The associated muscle atrophy after BoNT-A would seem a high price to pay in a disorder typified by weakness as a major determinant of motor dysfunction.

HOW DOES MUSCLE-TENDON LENGTHENING SURGERY AFFECT MUSCLE FUNCTION?

There are few studies on the effect of muscle-lengthening surgery on gross muscle architecture and function and currently no studies investigating the effect of surgery on sarcomere dynamics or other subcellular aspects of the function of the myofiber in CP. The available architectural studies, performed using ultrasound imaging, reveal large changes in muscle structure after surgery. Shortland et al. (2004) demonstrated a reduction of fascicle length of 25% in the medial gastrocnemius and an increase in pennation of 20%. Similarly, Haberfehlner et al. (2018) found a 30% reduction in semitendinosus length after medial hamstring surgery. Since semitendinosus is a long-fibered muscle, it is likely that its length reduction was due to fascicle shortening.

Perhaps the most likely cause of the observed reductions in fascicle length in these studies was due to a loss of sarcomeres. However, the alternative and intriguing possibility is that surgery results in a normalization (i.e. shortening) of sarcomere length (one recalls the reports of elongated sarcomeres in CP). Lichtwark and colleagues (2018) have used optical microendoscopy to measure sarcomere lengths in vivo in typically developing children demonstrating proximal-to-distal variation in sarcomere length in the tibialis anterior. It may be possible to perform similar measurements longitudinally in children with CP, answering important questions about the development of deformity and the impact of surgery.

FUTURE DIRECTION FOR CP MUSCLE RESEARCH

In this chapter, we have discussed important deficits in muscle structure at the gross, cellular, and molecular levels in children with CP, including reductions in muscle size, elongation of sarcomere length, and changes in the expression of titin. These extraordinary adaptations require further investigation with fundamental studies of early muscle development, particularly with regard to the possible influences of methylation and altered muscle innervation after cerebral injury, and to the effects of existing interventions. We believe that normalization of muscle function in early life by modifying early developmental processes may lead to more normal muscle growth during childhood and significant improvements in mobility of people with CP.

5-YEAR PRIORITIES

- Human studies investigating the role of satellite cells, connective tissue, sarcomeres, and titin on CP muscle growth and function to help guide the most appropriate treatment strategies.
- Development of novel, non-invasive treatments for CP muscle contracture which decrease muscle stiffness while preserving strength.
- Human studies quantifying the effects of BoNT-A on CP muscle to corroborate the sustained muscle atrophy and increased fibrofatty infiltration reported in animal studies.
- Further studies in DNA methylation of skeletal muscle – in particular, satellite cells – to help identify the cause of decreased sarcomerogenesis and fixed contracture in CP.
- In vivo human studies investigating the effect of muscle lengthening surgery on sarcomere mechanics and function.
- Development and application of early screening technologies – such as DNA methylation in peripheral blood – to allow for treatment with novel disease-modifying agents that improve muscle growth and function in children with CP.

REFERENCES

Albright AL, Cervi A, Singletary J (1991) Intrathecal baclofen for spasticity in cerebral palsy. *JAMA* **265**: 1418–1422.

Alhusaini AA, Crosbie J, Shepherd RB, Dean CM, Scheinberg A (2011) No change in calf muscle passive stiffness after botulinum toxin injection in children with cerebral palsy. *Dev Med Child Neurol* **53**: 553–558.

Alnaqeeb MA, Al Zaid NS, Goldspink G (1984) Connective tissue changes and physical properties of developing and aging skeletal muscle. *J Anat* **139**: 677–689.

Bartlett DJ, Hanna SE, Avery L, Stevenson RD, Galuppi B (2010) Correlates of decline in gross motor capacity in adolescents with cerebral palsy in Gross Motor Function Classification System levels III to V: an exploratory study. *Dev Med Child Neurol* **52**: e155–60.

Blumetti FC, Belloti JC, Tamaoki MJS, Pinto JA (2019) Botulinum toxin type A in the treatment of lower limb spasticity in children with cerebral palsy (Review). *Cochrane Database of Systematic Reviews* **10**: CD001408.

Booth CM, Cortina-Borja MJ, Theologis TN (2001) Collagen accumulation in muscles of children with cerebral palsy and correlation with severity of spasticity. *Dev Med Child Neurol* **43**: 314–320.

Brunengraber LN, Jayes FL, Leppert PC (2014) Injectable Clostridium histolyticum collagenase as a potential treatment for uterine fibroids. *Reprod Sci* **21**: 1452–1459.

Clowry GJ (2007) The dependence of spinal cord development on corticospinal input and its significance in understanding and treating spastic cerebral palsy. *Neurosci Biobehav Rev* **31**: 1114–1124.

Cosgrove AP, Graham HK (1994) Botulinum toxin A prevents the development of contractures in the hereditary spastic mouse. *Dev Med Child Neurol* **36**: 379–385.

Crowgey EL, Marsh AG, Robinson KG, Yeager SK, Akins RE (2018) Epigenetic machine learning: utilizing DNA methylation patterns to predict spastic cerebral palsy. *BMC Bioinformatics* **19**: 225

Dayanidhi S, Lieber RL (2014) Skeletal muscle satellite cells: Mediators of muscle growth during development and implications for developmental disorders. *Muscle Nerve* **50**: 723–732.

de Bruin M, Smeulders MJ, Kreulen M, Huijing PA, Jaspers RT (2014) Intramuscular connective tissue differences in spastic and control muscle: a mechanical and histological study. *PLoS One* **9**: e101038.

Fortuna R, Horisberger M, Vaz MA, Herzog W (2013) Do skeletal muscle properties recover following repeat onabotulinum toxin A injections? *J Biomech* **46**: 2426–2433.

Fortuna R, Vaz MA, Sawatsky A, Hart DA, Herzog W (2015) A clinically relevant BTX-A injection protocol leads to persistent weakness, contractile material loss, and an altered mRNA expression phenotype in rabbit quadriceps muscles. *J Biomech* **48**: 1700–1706.

Fortuna R, Vaz MA, Youssef AR, Longino D, Herzog W (2011) Changes in contractile properties of muscles receiving repeat injections of botulinum toxin (Botox). *J Biomech* **44**: 39–44.

Gillies AR, Lieber RL (2011) Structure and function of the skeletal muscle extracellular matrix. *Muscle Nerve* **44**: 318–331.

Gim JA, Hong CP, Kim DS et al. (2015) Genome-Wide Analysis of DNA Methylation before- and after Exercise in the Thoroughbred Horse with MeDIP-Seq. *Mol. Cells* **38**: 210–220.

Gordon AM, Huxley AF, Julian FJ (1966) The variation in isometric tension with sarcomere length in vertebrate muscle fibres. *J Physiol* **184**: 170–192.

Gose S, Sakai T, Shibata T, Murase T, Yoshikawa H, Sugamoto K (2010) Morphometric Analysis of the Femur in Cerebral Palsy: 3-dimensional CT Study. *J Pediatr Orthop* **30**: 568–574.

Gough M, Fairhurst C, Shortland AP (2005) Botulinum toxin and cerebral palsy: time for reflection? *Dev Med Child Neurol* **47**: 709–712.

Gough M, Shortland AP (2012) Could muscle deformity in children with spastic cerebral palsy be related to an impairment of muscle growth and altered adaptation? *Dev Med Child Neurol* **54**: 495–499.

Graham HK. Cerebral Palsy. (2014) In: Lovell WW, Winter RB editors, *Lovell and Winter's Pediatric Orthopaedics, 7th Ed*. Philadelphia: Lippincott Williams & Wilkins.

Graham HK, Boyd R, Carlin JB et al. (2008) Does botulinum toxin a combined with bracing prevent hip displacement in children with cerebral palsy and "hips at risk"? A randomized, controlled trial. *J Bone Joint Surg Am* **90**: 23–33.

Graham HK, Rosenbaum P, Paneth N et al. (2016) Cerebral palsy. *Nat Rev Dis Primers* **2**: 15082.

Graham HK, Selber P (2003) Musculoskeletal aspects of cerebral palsy *J Bone Joint Surg Br* **85**: 157–166.

Haberfehlner H, Jaspers RT, Rutz E et al. (2018) Outcome of medial hamstring lengthening in children with spastic paresis: A biomechanical and morphological observational study. *PLoS One* **13**: e0192573.

Hartley I, Elkhoury FF, Heon Shin J et al. (2013) Long-lasting changes in DNA methylation following short-term hypoxic exposure in primary hippocampal neuronal cultures. *PLoS One* **8**: e77859.

Hasnat MJ, Rice JE (2015) Intrathecal baclofen for treating spasticity in children with cerebral palsy. *Cochrane Database Syst Rev* **13**: CD004552.

Herskind A, Ritterband-Rosenbaum A, Willerslev-Olsen M et al. (2016). Muscle growth is reduced in 15-month-old children with cerebral palsy. *Dev Med Child Neurol* **58**: 485–491.

Herzog W (2014) The role of titin in eccentric muscle contraction. *J Exp Biol* **217**: 2825–2833.

Hof AL (2001) Changes in muscles and tendons due to neural motor disorders: implications for therapeutic intervention. *Neural Plast* **8**: 71–81.

Houtepen LC, Vinkers CH, Carrillo-Roa T et al. (2016) Genome-wide DNA methylation levels and altered cortisol stress reactivity following childhood trauma in humans. *Nat Commun* **7**: 10967.

Howard JJ, Khot A, Graham HK (2019) The hip in cerebral palsy. In: Alshyrda S, Howard JJ, Huntley JS, Schoenecker J, editors. *The Pediatric and Adolescent Hip: Essentials and Evidence*. Switzerland: Springer.

Howard JJ, Huntley JS, Graham HK, Herzog W (2019) Intramuscular Injection of Collagenase Clostridium Histolyticum May Decrease Spastic Muscle Contracture for Children with Cerebral Palsy. *Med Hypotheses* **122**: 126–128.

Howard JJ, Soo B, Graham HK et al. (2005) Cerebral palsy in Victoria: Motor types, topography and gross motor function. *J Paediatr Child Health* **41**: 479–483.

Huntley JS, Bradley LJ (2017) The evidence base for botulinum toxin injection for the treatment of cerebral palsy-related spasticity in the lower limb: the long-term effects. In: Alshyrda S, Huntley JS, Banaszkiewicz PA, editors. *Paediatric Orthopaedics: An Evidence-Based Approach to Clinical Questions*. Switzerland: Springer Nature, pp 369–373.

Hurst LC, Badalamente MA, Hentz VR et al. (2009) Injectable collagenase clostridium histolyticum for Dupuytren's contracture. *N Eng J Med* **361**: 968–979.

Huxley AF, Niedergerke R (1954) Structural changes in muscle during contraction; interference microscopy of living muscle fibres. *Nature* **173**: 971–973.

Kalsi G, Fry NR, Shortland AP (2016) Gastrocnemius muscle-tendon interaction during walking in typically-developing adults and children, and in children with spastic cerebral palsy. *J Biomech* **49**: 3194–3199.

Koman LA, Mooney JF 3rd, Smith B, Goodman A, Mulvaney T (1993) Management of cerebral palsy with botulinum-A toxin: preliminary investigation. *J Pediatr Orthop* **13**: 489–495.

Labeit D, Watanabe K, Witt C et al. (2003) Calcium-dependent molecular spring elements in the giant protein titin. *Proc Natl Acad Sci U S A* **100**: 13716–13721.

Larkin-Kaiser KS, Howard JJ, Leonard TR et al. (2019) Relationship Of Muscle Morphology And Hip Displacement In Spastic Cerebral Palsy: A Pilot Study Investigating Changes Intrinsic to the Sarcomere. *J Orthop Surg Res* **14**: 187.

Larson JE, Snyder B (2019) The hip in spinal muscular atrophy. In: Alshyrda S, Howard JJ, Huntley JS, Schoenecker J, editors. *The Pediatric and Adolescent Hip: Essentials and Evidence*. Switzerland: Springer.

Lee KM, Kang JY, Chung CY et al. (2010) Clinical Relevance of Valgus Deformity of Proximal Femur in Cerebral Palsy. *J Pediatr Orthop* **30**: 720–725.

Lee S, Dabney K, Sees J, Miller F, Shrader W, Akins R (2019) Atypical populations of muscle satellite cells are associated with spastic cerebral palsy [abstract]. *Dev Med Child Neurol* **61**: 64.

Leonard TR, Howard J, Larkin-Kaiser K et al. (2019) Stiffness of hip adductor myofibrils is decreased in children with spastic cerebral palsy. *J Biomech* **87**: 100–106.

Levine LA, Schmid TM, EmeighHart SG, Tittelbach T, McLane MP, Tursi JP (2014) Collagenase clostridium histolyticum degrades type I and III collagen while sparing type IV collagen in vitro in Peyronie's plaque explants [abstract no PD22-03 plus oral presentation], *American Urological Association Annual Meeting*. Orlando: American Urological Association Annual Meeting.

Lichtwark GA, Farris DJ, Chen X, Hodges PW, Delp SL (2018) Microendoscopy reveals positive correlation in multiscale length changes and variable sarcomere lengths across different regions of human muscle. *J Appl Physiol* **125**: 1812–1820.

Lynn AK, Turner M, Chambers HG (2009) Surgical management of spasticity in persons with cerebral palsy. *PM R* **1**: 834–838.

Miller F, Dabney KW, Rang M (1995) Complications in Cerebral Palsy Treatment. In: Epps CH Jr, Bowen JR, editors, *Complications in Pediatric Orthopedic Surgery*. Philadelphia: Lippincott-Raven Publishers, pp 477–544.

Miller SD, Juricic M, Hesketh K et al. (2017) Prevention of hip displacement in children with cerebral palsy: a systematic review. *Dev Med Child Neurol* **59**: 1130–1139.

Minamoto VB, Suzuki KP, Bremner S, Lieber RL, Ward SR (2015) Dramatic Changes in Muscle Contractile and Structural Properties After Two Botulinum Toxin Injections. *Muscle Nerve* **52**: 649–657.

Molenaers G, Desloovere K, Fabry G, De Cock P (2006) The Effects of Quantitative Gait Assessment and Botulinum Toxin A on Musculoskeletal Surgery in Children with Cerebral Palsy. *J Bone Joint Surg* **88**: 161–169.

Multani I, Manji J, Tang MJ, Herzog W, Howard JJ, Graham HK (2019) Sarcopenia, Cerebral Palsy and Botulinum Toxin A. *JBJS Reviews* **7**: e4.

Noble JJ, Fry NR, Lewis AP, Keevil SF, Gough M, Shortland AP (2013) Lower limb muscle volumes in bilateral spastic cerebral palsy. *Brain Dev* **36**: 294–300.

Novak I, McIntyre S, Morgan C, et al. (2013) A systematic review of interventions for children with cerebral palsy: state of the evidence. *Dev Med Child Neurol* **55**: 885–910.

Phelps WM (1959) Prevention of acquired dislocation of the hip in cerebral palsy. J Bone Joint Surg Am **41**: 440–448.

Pingel J, Bartels EM, Nielsen J (2017a) New perspectives on the development of muscle contractures following central motor lesions. *J Physiol* **595**: 1027–1038.

Pingel J, Nielsen MS, Lauridsen T et al. (2017b) Injection of high dose botulinum-toxin A leads to impaired skeletal muscle function and damage of the fibrilar and non-fibrilar structures. *Sci Rep* **7**: 14746.

Pingel J, Wienecke J, Lorentzen J, Nielsen JB (2016) Botulinum toxin injection causes hyperreflexia and increased muscle stiffness of the triceps surae muscle in the rat. *J Neurophysiol* **116**: 2615–2623.

Rang M (1990) Cerebral Palsy. In: Lovell WW, Winter RB eds. *Lovell and Winter's Pediatric Orthopaedics, 7th Ed.* Philadelphia: Lippincott Williams & Wilkins.

Robin J, Graham HK, Selber P, Dobson F, Smith K, Baker R (2008) Proximal femoral geometry in cerebral palsy: a population-based cross-sectional study. *J Bone Joint Surg Br* **90**: 1372–1379.

Robinson K, Crowgey E, Marsh A, Lee S, Akins R (2019) Altered gene expression and DNA methylation profiles in skeletal muscle from individuals with spastic CP [abstract]. *Dev Med Child Neurol* **61**: 51.

Schless SH, Cenni F, Bar-On L et al. (2018) Medial gastrocnemius volume and echo-intensity after botulinum neurotoxin A interventions in children with spastic cerebral palsy. *Dev Med Child Neurol* **61**: 783–790.

Seaborne RA, Strauss J, Cocks M et al. (2018) Human Skeletal Muscle Possesses an Epigenetic Memory of Hypertrophy. *Sci Rep* **8**: 1898.

Sharples AP, Stewart CE, Seaborne RA (2016) Does skeletal muscle have an 'epi'-memory? The role of epigenetics in nutritional programming, metabolic disease, aging and exercise. *Aging Cell* **15**: 603–616.

Shortland AP, Fry NR, Eve LC, Gough M (2004) Changes to medial gastrocnemius architecture after surgical intervention in spastic diplegia. *Dev Med Child Neurol* **46**: 667–673.

Smith LR, Chambers HG, Lieber RL (2013) Reduced satellite cell population may lead to contractures in children with cerebral palsy. *Dev Med Child Neurol* **55**: 264–270.

Smith LR, Lee KS, Ward SR, Chambers HG, Lieber RL (2011) Hamstring contractures in children with spastic cerebral palsy result from a stiffer extracellular matrix and increased in vivo sarcomere length. *J Physiol* **589**: 2625–2639.

Soo B, Howard JJ, Boyd RN et al. (2006) Hip displacement in cerebral palsy. *J Bone Joint Surg Am* **88**: 121–129.

Tachdjian MO, Minear WL (1956) Hip dislocation in cerebral palsy. *J Bone Joint Surg Am* **38**: 1358–1364.

Tedroff K, Granath F, Forssberg H, Haglund-Akerlind Y (2009) Long-term effects of botulinum toxin A in children with cerebral palsy. *Dev Med Child Neurol* **51**: 120–127.

Tedroff K, Hägglund G, Miller F (2019) Long-term effects of selective dorsal rhizotomy in children with cerebral palsy: a systematic review. *Dev Med Child Neurol* **62**: 554–562

Tedroff K, Löwing K, Åström E (2015) A prospective cohort study investigating gross motor function, pain, and health-related quality of life 17 years after selective dorsal rhizotomy in cerebral palsy. *Dev Med Child Neurol* **57**: 484–490.

Tedroff K, Löwing K, Jacobson D, Åström E (2011) Does loss of spasticity matter? A 10-year follow-up after selective dorsal rhizotomy in cerebral palsy. *Dev Med Child Neurol* **53**: 724–729.

Wang KK, Munger ME, Chen BP, Novacheck TF (2018) Selective dorsal rhizotomy in ambulant children with cerebral palsy. *J Child Orthop* **12**: 413–427.

Willoughby K, Ang SG, Thomason P, Graham HK (2012) The impact of botulinum toxin A and abduction bracing on long-term development in children with cerebral palsy. *Dev Med Child Neurol* **54**: 743–747.

Yam WK, Leung MS (2006) Interrater reliability of Modified Ashworth Scale and Modified Tardieu Scale in children with spastic cerebral palsy. *J Child Neurol* **21**: 1031–1035.

Yin H, Price F, Rudnicki MA (2013) Satellite cells and the muscle stem cell niche. *Physiol Rev* **93**: 23–67.

Treatment of Muscle-Tendon Unit Dysfunction in Children with Cerebral Palsy:

Historical Overview, Current Practices, and Impact of Physics-based Modeling

Jon R Davids, Anahid Ebrahimi, and Darryl G Thelen

KEY POINTS

- Myostatic contractures of the muscle-tendon unit (MTU) are common in children with cerebral palsy, with muscle function further compromised by impairments of spasticity and selective motor control.
- Current soft tissue surgical treatments of contractures seek to minimize muscle weakness following lengthening of the MTU.
- Physics based models provide a framework for investigating soft tissue treatments and are most impactful when the models have a solid biomechanical foundation and are supported by objective metrics.

OPPORTUNITIES

- Well formulated models and more objective data are needed to continue to question traditional dogma and consider factors that remain beyond the scope of conventional clinical treatment considerations.
- Advances in imaging, modeling, and sensors of dynamic muscle behavior should enable more objective planning of soft tissue treatments.
- Intraoperative sensors and better knowledge translation practices could enhance the precision with which soft tissue treatments are performed and improve consistency across surgeons and institutions.

HISTORICAL OVERVIEW

From the early 1950s through to the 1970s, decision making and technical execution of surgery to improve gait in children with cerebral palsy (CP) was based upon previous clinical experience in the management of children with polio (Rang, JLovell, and Winter 1986). This attempted carryover of surgical management strategy between disease processes was based upon the recognition that the clinical manifestations of both diseases included similar gait deviations, muscle weakness, and fixed contractures of muscle-tendon units (MTU). However, there were distinct elements of disease pathophysiology that would prove to have significant impacts on the outcomes following soft tissue surgeries designed for patients with polio when applied to children with CP.

Polio, short for poliomyelitis, or infantile paralysis, is an infectious disease caused by the poliovirus. Ancient Egyptian documents describe crippling diseases compatible with polio. Outbreaks of polio in resource-rich countries in the Northern Hemisphere, typically occurring in the summer and fall, and have been reported since the mid-19th century. In the 20th century, polio epidemics became increasingly severe. The increasing age of persons affected by primary infection was associated with increasing disease severity and subsequent impairment and/or death. Polio reached its peak in the United States in 1952, with more than 21 000 paralytic cases. Fortunately, following the introduction of effective vaccines, polio incidences rapidly declined (Oshinsky 2006). Although the last case of wild-type polio virus infection acquired in the United States was in 1979, global eradication of polio remains an elusive goal (Center for Disease Control and Prevention 2005).

The poliovirus enters through the mouth, and primary multiplication of the virus occurs at the site of implantation in the pharynx and gastrointestinal tract. The virus invades local lymphoid tissue, enters the bloodstream, and then may infect the cells of the central nervous system. Replication of poliovirus in motor neurons of the anterior horn and brain stem leads to inflammation and cell destruction, resulting in the typical manifestations of polio. Associated impairment of the specifically innervated muscles ranges from weakness to complete flaccid paralysis (Center for Disease Control and Prevention 2005). Long-term motor imbalance in a growing child results in joint contractures, the development of fixed or myostatic shortening of the MTU, and progressive skeletal deformities. Unaffected muscles retain normal strength, tone, and selective motor control.

CP refers to a group of neurological disorders that appear in infancy or early childhood and permanently affect body movement and muscle coordination (Rosenbaum et al. 2007). CP is caused by damage to or structural abnormalities of the developing brain that disrupts the brain's ability to control movement and maintain posture and balance. CP is currently considered the most common cause of childhood disability, with a prevalence of 3.3 children per 1000 live births, and appears to be unchanged over the last 60 years (Oskoui et al. 2013). Regardless of whether the cause is acquired or developed, the damage is non-repairable, and the impairments that result are permanent. While the abnormality of the central nervous system is described as being static (i.e. unchanging) in the great majority of children with CP, symptoms differ in type and severity from one person to the next, and the clinical manifestations may change with the child's growth and development. In addition to motor impairments, individuals with CP may have some level of intellectual disability, seizures, impaired vision, diminished hearing, and speech problems (Rosenbaum et al. 2007).

Dysfunctions and deformities of the MTU in children with CP are sequential and progressive. Young children with CP may exhibit weakness, increased muscle tone, and diminished selective control of the muscle, but the resting length of the MTU is typical for age. With growth and development, fixed shortening or contracture of the MTU (myostatic deformity) may occur. In addition, long-term motor imbalance in a growing child results in the development of joint contractures and progressive skeletal deformities.

The clinical phenotypes of children with either polio or CP include muscle weakness and myostatic contractures of the MTU. Function of the MTU in children with CP is further compromised by impairments of spasticity and selective motor control. Surgical treatments of soft tissue deformities carried over from polio to CP focused on releasing or aggressive lengthening of the MTU to restore range of motion.

Clinical decision making for surgery to improve gait for children with CP, and outcome assessment following surgery, were based upon non-standardized observational gait analysis and tabletop physical examination and assessment of range of motion.

In the early 1980s, development and application of computer-based quantitative gait analysis (QGA) began to provide objective evidence that the outcomes following surgery based upon this paradigm were unpredictable, and in some cases, actually detrimental. Application of biomechanical principles improved the understanding of gait disruption in children with CP by recognizing the function of a muscle during gait is to generate a moment, which is influenced by the muscle's ability to generate force, and the distance that this force is applied from the joint's center of rotation (lever arm). Subsequent studies established that children with CP were weaker than typically developing peers, and that strength training, which had previously been thought to worsen function by exacerbating spasticity, could actually have a positive effect on muscle function during gait (Mockford and Caulton 2008; Wiley and Damiano 2008). This led to the development of the concept of a strength-to-weight ratio that became progressively less favorable to independent ambulation as children proceeded into adolescence and adulthood (Davids et al. 2014). It was also established that aggressive surgical lengthening of the MTU resulted in additional weakness that, in some cases, resulted in the development of additional gait deviations that further compromised gait function (Firth et al. 2013).

By the 1990s, these realizations led to the development of new clinical decision making paradigms that relied heavily on the data generated by QGA, emphasizing early tone management and surgical correction of skeletal lever arm dysfunction (Narayanan 2012; Graham et al. 2016). Subsequently, new surgical techniques, based upon improved understanding of the pathoanatomy and pathophysiology of muscle in individuals with spasticity, were developed for correcting myostatic deformity of the MTU (Tinney et al. 2014; Davids et al. 2019). These techniques were designed to result in less weakness of the MTU following surgical lengthening. Improvements in anaesthetic techniques and peri-surgical pain management allowed for simultaneous surgical correction of all primary musculoskeletal problems causing gait deviations (single-event multilevel surgery [SEMLS]). The importance of proper rehabilitation to regain muscle strength following these surgeries has also been appreciated (Seniorou et al. 2007).

CURRENT SURGICAL PRACTICES FOR SOFT TISSUE TREATMENT

Current understanding of the pathoanatomy of myostatic deformity of the MTU in children with CP recognizes that the tendon is relatively longer, the muscle belly is relatively shorter, and the muscle fiber is relatively longer (or stretched) when compared to typically developing peers (Shortland et al. 2009; Barrett and Lichtwark 2010). Tenotomy or complete release of the MTU at its insertion into bone results in excessive weakness and should, therefore, be avoided. Surgical techniques that lengthen through the muscle belly are too destructive to the MTU's contractile components and should never be used when performing surgery to improve gait. Surgical lengthening at the anatomical transition from muscle belly to tendon (by either intramuscular tenotomy or fractional lengthening of the aponeurosis, depending on the architecture of the targeted MTU) has been shown by muscle modeling and clinical studies to achieve controlled lengthening of the MTU while minimizing subsequent weakness (Delp, Statler, and Carroll 1995; Dreher et al. 2012; Firth et al. 2013).

An animal model study of fractional lengthening of the aponeurosis has shown effective lengthening of the MTU, with shortening of the muscle fibers at and distal to the level of the aponeurectomy (Jaspers et al. 2005). In this setting, shortening (or relaxing) of the long (stretched) muscle fibers could result in improvement at the location on the length-tension curve at the sarcomere level. These findings suggest that optimally executed lengthening of the MTU at the level of the aponeurosis could result in an improved strength profile for the targeted muscle. A recent study confirmed these theoretical observations, showing maintenance of isometric strength, and improved isokinetic strength of knee flexion following surgical lengthening of the medial hamstring muscles (Davids et al. 2019). In properly selected patients, who receive optimally executed surgery, followed by appropriate rehabilitation (orthotics and physical therapy), weakness following surgical lengthening of the MTU is not inevitable.

The SEMLS paradigm for soft tissue surgery to improve gait in children with CP is based upon the development of best practices in six areas (Davids et al. 2004). Clinical decision-making is based upon a diagnostic matrix that integrates data from the clinical history, physical examination, diagnostic imaging, QGA, and examination under anaesthesia. (1) New patient-reported tools and a broader framework for assessment of impairment and disability have improved the quality and relevance of information gained from patient histories. (2) Improved precision and interpretation of QGA data has diminished (but not completely replaced) the significance of the examination under anaesthesia in the diagnostic matrix. (3) Surgical techniques for soft tissue surgery focus on lengthening at the myotendinous junction of the MTU and are designed to minimize the possibility of over lengthening, which results in excessive weakness. (4) Pain management is proactive, utilizing a combination of narcotic and anti-inflammatory medications, delivered centrally, regionally, or locally to minimize the pain associated with aggressive SEMLS surgery. Optimal tone management greatly facilitates pain management at all stages following soft tissue surgery in children with CP. (5) Postsurgical rehabilitation requires intensive community-based physical therapy for 4 to 8 months following SEMLS surgery. (6) Orthotic management is an integral element of rehabilitation following SEMLS surgery (Davids, Rowan, and Davis 2007). A relatively restrictive orthotic design (i.e. a solid ankle-foot orthosis) protects soft tissue healing immediately following surgery and compensates for early weakness. Conversion to a less restrictive design (i.e. posterior leaf spring orthotic) is usually appropriate 4 to 6 months following surgery.

Outcome assessment in body structure and function domains is best achieved by utilizing QGA at regular intervals following SEMLS surgery. Assessment of outcomes in activity and participation domains is currently best accomplished through patient-reported outcomes tools. Future assessment of outcomes in these domains may be enhanced by the development of wearable movement measurement technologies that facilitate the quantitative assessment during community-based events.

ROLE OF MODELS IN GUIDING AND EVALUATING SOFT TISSUE TREATMENTS

Musculoskeletal models provide a framework to investigate the underlying causes of gait disorders and to gain insights into treatment options. A typical model includes a linked segment representation of the human body with musculotendon actuators acting about joints of the lower extremities (Fig. 9.1). Models are often used in biomechanics to estimate internal soft tissue loads that cannot be directly measured or to explore 'what if' scenarios (Robertson et al. 2013). The earliest models for estimating muscle and joint contact forces appeared in the literature around 50 years ago (Seireg and Arvikar 1973 and 1975). Since then, models have evolved in complexity as imaging and experimental capabilities have improved to provide better data, and improved computational resources and software to address more complex problems.

Musculoskeletal models can generally be solved by taking one of two approaches: 'top-down' or 'bottom-up' (Vaughan, Davis, and O'Connor 1992). The 'top-down' approach considers the actuation of movement as it occurs in reality – the brain sends a signal through the central nervous system, which excites the muscles and induces movement about the joints. This is modeled as a forward dynamics simulation, in which the muscle excitations are the inputs to the model and result in the predicted motion of the body. Alternatively, inverse dynamics modeling takes a 'bottom-up' approach, using measures of external kinematics and forces to ascertain the joint kinematics and kinetic patterns. When coupled with a musculoskeletal representation, one can also estimate the underlying musculotendon lengths and velocities. However, the muscle redundancy problem must be solved to estimate individual muscle forces that generate measured joint torques. Numerical optimization (Seireg and Arvikar 1975) and/or electromyographic (EMG) recordings (Thelen 2003) are the most common approach to solving this indeterminate problem, but muscle force estimates obtained with either approach come with a degree of uncertainty (Erdemir et al. 2007) and can be particularly circumspect when applied to pathological cases such as a patient with CP. As a result, most gait labs typically only report joint angles, joint kinetics, EMG, and (sometimes) muscle-tendon kinematics when analyzing individual gait disorders. Of these measures, the greatest amount of information for treatment planning is gleaned from gait kinematics. This preference is consistent with the fact that kinematics are the gauge by which the effectiveness of a treatment is often evaluated.

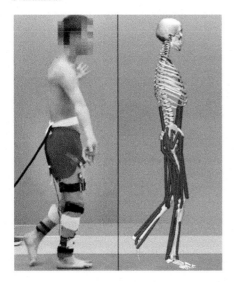

Figure 9.1 Physics-based models describe the relationship between neural excitation, muscle actuation, and dynamic movement. Such models are used to estimate kinematics and loading of soft tissue and provide a framework to investigate mechanistic causes and treatment of gait disorders. Image of model taken from OpenSim Software reprinted, with permission, from Delp et al. 2007 © 2007 IEEE.

There has long been hope that predictive (forward dynamic) musculoskeletal simulations would become sophisticated enough to be used in clinical treatment of gait disorders. In such a scenario, an individual would come into a motion analysis laboratory, undergo physical examination, medical imaging, and gait analysis. A model representing the individual's musculoskeletal geometry would then be created. Simulations of that model would be generated that predict the individual's pathological gait pattern. One could then simulate orthopedic and conservative treatment options and then could predict how the individual would walk post-treatment. Such a vision parallels the use of computational modeling in many engineering fields, where virtual experiments are often relied upon to make design decisions. There have been recent attempts to implement such an approach and evaluate predictions on case studies (Pitto et al. 2019). However, there remain many uncertainties in these complex models, including uncertain soft tissue properties, simplifications in muscle-tendon geometry mechanics, and assumed representations of neural control. Hence, physics-based gait simulation models remain insufficient to guide patient-specific treatment. Alternatively, musculoskeletal models are well suited to conducting thought experiments, thereby providing a framework for generating testable hypotheses and interpreting empirical observations.

For clinical purposes, the most useful models address a fundamental mechanical question that underlies the basis for treatment. To be effective, the models should be transparent with respect to assumptions, and the output of the models should be clear and sufficiently easy to understand and/or apply. It is recognized that acceptance among clinicians is easier when the study results are consistent with observations on patients' experience and intuition. However, acceptance is more difficult when results are apparently inconsistent with clinical dogma and/or experience. In these cases, there is a better chance of acceptance when there is equipoise concerning the clinical question, and the model has solid biomechanical foundation. While full validation is generally not achievable, demonstrating consistency between predictions and empirical observations is key to enhance confidence in results (Hicks et al. 2015). The following are some historical examples of modeling papers that have effectively bridged the gap between modeling, clinical treatments, and observations in CP gait disorders.

How should plantar flexor contractures be treated? In 1994, Delp and colleagues conducted a modeling study to compare the effects of aponeurosis and Achilles tendon lengthening on plantar flexor strength and range of motion (Delp, Statler, and Carroll 1995). Prior clinical studies had found that Achilles tendon lengthening procedures for coupled gastrocnemius and soleus contractures had negative ramifications on strength (Sharrard and Bernstein 1972; Rose et al. 1993). Musculoskeletal simulations showed that Achilles tendon lengthening is not effective in accounting for differences in the architecture of the triceps surae muscles. In contrast, an aponeurosis lengthening during an isolated gastrocnemius contracture was effective in both relieving the contracture and returning the torque generating characteristics of the plantar flexor. The results provided a theoretical construct for understanding clinical results and a clinical preference away from Achilles tendon lengthening due to the adverse effects on plantar flexor strength.

Who are good candidates for hamstring lengthening? Crouch gait was long attributed to excessively 'short' or 'spastic' hamstrings that restrict knee extension, an abnormality that could be corrected through surgical lengthening (DeLuca et al. 1998). Musculoskeletal models and gait analysis data were subsequently used to investigate the veracity of this explanation. Surprisingly, early studies showed that the hamstrings often do not act at abnormally short lengths in individuals walking with a crouch gait (Delp et al. 1996). Follow-up outcome studies found that hamstring lengthening may not always be appropriate in children with CP who have neither short nor abnormally slow hamstring MTUs (Arnold et al. 2006). In such cases, the lengthening procedure can result in unsatisfactory knee extension and/or anterior pelvic tilt. This study has led to some labs using model-based estimates of hamstring lengths and velocities to identify candidates for hamstring lengthening procedures.

What are the implications of patellar advancement in baja? Patellar tendon advancement (PTA) is often recommended for children with CP who have quadriceps insufficiency, defined as an inability to actively extend the knee. PTA involves surgically moving the patellar tendon insertion inferiorly and is often coupled with a distal femoral extension osteotomy (DEFO) to treat crouch gait. Musculoskeletal models have been used to investigate the biomechanical ramifications of the standard PTA procedure, which moves the patella from an abnormally superior (alta) to a posterior position (baja) (Stout et al. 2008). Musculoskeletal models have shown that patella alta actually enhances the patellar tendon moment arm in a flexed posture, and hence may beneficially diminish quadriceps forces for individuals walking in crouch (Lenhart et al. 2017). Surgical placement in patella baja can enhance moment arms in an extended posture and thus may be beneficial if crouch is fully resolved. A subsequent retrospective study of radiographic images found evidence of enhanced patellar tendon moment arms after DEFO together with PTA procedures that were consistent with model predictions (Fig. 9.2) (Bittmann et al. 2018). However, these modeling studies revealed that baja reduces patellar tendon moment arms in more flexed postures, and thereby may compromise strength in flexed knee tasks such as sit-to-stand and stair climbing. The modeling work led to an evaluation of sit-to-stand abilities in individuals who previously underwent coupled DFEO+PTA, which did indeed find evidence of knee extensor dysfunction. The DFEO+PTA group required more time to stand and absorbed less knee power. These observations have raised the question of whether less aggressive advancement of the patella may improve sit-to-stand function without compromising short- and long-term gait improvements that have been observed using the conventional PTA procedure.

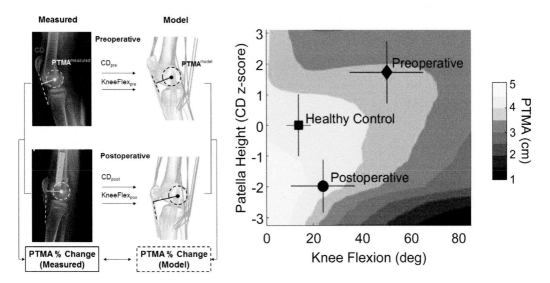

Figure 9.2 (LEFT) Models and radiographs demonstrate the enhanced patellar tendon moment arm (PTMA) achieved in an extended posture via patellar tendon advancement (PTA). (RIGHT) However, the placement of the patella in baja may diminish the PTMA relative to healthy controls in flexed knee postures. This may have implications on functional performance in functional tasks, e.g. sit-to-stand, involving large substantial knee flexion. Reprinted from Bittmann et al. 2018 with permission from Elsevier.

The previous examples demonstrate the potential to use models to provide insights relevant for making and understanding the ramifications of treatment decisions in gait disorders. There remain many opportunities for using models to question traditional dogma or consider factors that remain beyond the scope of conventional clinical treatment considerations and address many open questions in the treatment of CP gait disorders. As an example, it has recently been shown that muscle spindle firing rates during passive stretch exhibit a direct dependence on force (Blum et al. 2017), rather than the traditionally presumed dependence on length and velocity. Mathematical descriptions of the force-dependent stretch response have since been incorporated into musculoskeletal models, which can predict characteristic limb motion during the pendulum test in children with spastic CP (De Groote et al. 2018). Further, it has recently been shown that a spasticity model based on feedback from muscle force can better predict spurious EMG activity during walking in children with CP than spasticity models that only consider muscle length and velocity (Falisse et al. 2018). Such modeling work is important because it provides a causal framework to re-evaluate conventional perspectives of spasticity and may provide an improved perspective by which to interpret EMG measurements in gait.

Another opportunity to use modeling is in consideration of gait treatments on joint tissue loading and health. In the field of osteoarthritis, cartilage tissue loading is often linked as a factor contributing to early-onset joint degeneration and osteoarthritis. Many treatments for gait disorders introduce disruptive changes in cartilage tissue loading that could have the same ramifications for joint health. Advances in image-based musculoskeletal models and solution techniques are opening avenues to simulate how orthopedic treatments for CP gait disorders affect joint tissue loading. For example, a model of the PTA procedure illustrates the spurious cartilage loading patterns that can emerge if crouch gait is not resolved (Brandon et al. 2018) (Fig. 9.3). These results were obtained using a generic knee model of a typically developing patient. Advances in musculoskeletal imaging, segmentation techniques, and statistical shape modeling could enable one to consider altered skeletal geometry that often arises in CP. Such studies are warranted along with long-term follow-ups to ascertain whether orthopedic factors may predispose patients to early joint degeneration and osteoarthritis.

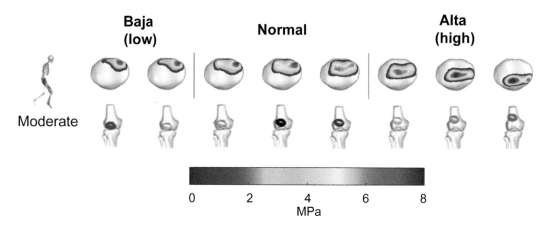

Figure 9.3 Patellofemoral contact pressures on a representative child with CP with moderate crouch gait and altered patellar position. Reprinted from Brandon et al. 2018, with permission from Elsevier.

5-YEAR GOALS

The advancements made in modeling have had a substantial impact on our understanding of muscle-tendon treatment in children with CP. However, clinical acceptance, as will be discussed at the end of this chapter, is slow. Much of the quantitative interpretation used in treatment planning is based on physical exam and gait kinematics rather than the underlying muscle activations and kinetics that drive the movement. This needs to evolve and allow for more precise planning and execution of soft tissue treatments. The following are three interrelated areas that could enable that to happen: (1) more comprehensive characterization of muscle-tendon behavior in pathological gait, (2) enhance precision in carrying out soft tissue treatments, and (3) generation of more outcomes data.

Our thought process for the 5 year goals parallels advances made in correcting bony deformities (Novacheck and Gage 2007; Schwartz, Rozumalski, and Novacheck 2014). Newer technology exists that can provide a 3D reconstruction of the bone deformity from images, and can identify appropriate cuts to reshape the bone into a desired geometry and then provide the surgeon with the hardware needed to precisely and efficiently carry out the procedure (Athwal et al. 2003). Ideally, a similar overall process would be available for soft tissue treatments. However, implementation is clearly more complex given the desired outcome, e.g. certain muscle behavior during walking, depends on geometry, neuromuscular control, and the behavior of the rest of the musculoskeletal system. There are historical, experiential-based clinical indications for specific soft tissue treatments. For example, algorithms exist for ascertaining whether an individual is a good candidate for a hamstring lengthening (Arnold et al. 2006). However, that decision process is based on a generic musculoskeletal model and does not inform the surgeon on how much to lengthen the hamstrings and is made more complex by the addition of concomitant procedures on whether you need to lengthen hamstrings simultaneously. There is potential for making these decisions more objective, precise, and more tightly linked to outcomes, but that requires more data, which we believe can be generated with newer technologies.

Current gait analysis laboratories provide measures of EMG activity and, sometimes, muscle-tendon kinematics. EMG is most commonly evaluated subjectively, whereas muscle-tendon kinematics are evaluated using suspect model assumptions. There are newer technologies that allow for better assessments of muscle control, kinematics, and kinetics, all of which should be evaluated when considering candidates for soft tissue treatment. Muscle synergy analysis approaches have emerged for characterizing selective motor control and are showing remarkable promise for predicting the outcomes of procedures (Schwartz, Rozumalski, and Steele 2016). Further development and extension of this metric across laboratories could enable more labs to use this approach. Generation of muscle-specific skeletal and joint geometry from images is becoming viable with better image segmentation technology based on machine learning techniques. These capabilities could enable one to better ascertain muscle lengths based on an individual's anatomy and thereby provide a more quantitative basis for identifying muscles that are too short and how much they should be lengthened by. Finally, it would be remiss to not recognize that many procedures are aimed at altering the force output of muscles during gait, making force a more relevant measure than length. The recent introduction of shear wave tensiometry may make it feasible to measure individual muscle-tendon forces in children with CP (Fig. 9.4) (Martin et al. 2018). Tensiometers use micron-scale taps to induce shear waves in tendons and in-series accelerometers to monitor the wave propagation speed, which provides a metric of force (Keuler et al. 2019). Tensiometers can record at rates up to $100Hz$ sufficient for studying human movement dynamics. The noninvasiveness and simplicity of this technology is particularly exciting given that it could be widely deployed. Taken together, we believe that better characterizations of muscle-tendon kinematics, kinetics, and controls could provide quantitative targets for the magnitude of changes to induce in soft tissue procedures such as transfers and lengthenings.

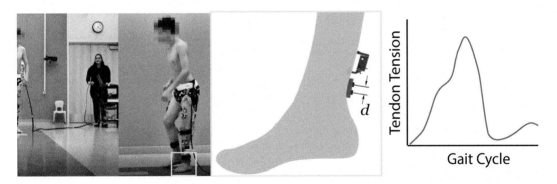

Figure 9.4 Shear wave tensiometers, shown placed on the participant's left limb patellar and Achilles tendons, can provide muscle-tendon force information during a standard gait analysis (left images). The shear wave tensiometer device (middle graphic) consists of a piezo-electric tapper and two accelerometers (red and blue) set a fixed distance (d) apart. Tendon tension can be estimated during dynamic tasks, like walking (right graph), based on its proportional relationship with shear wave speed (Martin et al. 2018). Figure adapted from Keuler et al. 2019 under Creative Commons CC BY license.

The next major challenge in soft tissue treatment is enhancing the precision with which treatments are carried out. For orthopedic treatments, this means having precise targets for correction and a means by which to carry it out. For example, tendon transfer may be defined to introduce a certain change in muscle length or lever arm about a joint. Medical images could be used to identify a precise target, and there could be guides generated to enable that to happen. For muscle lengthening procedures, precision is more challenging. Current aponeurosis based contracture-relief procedures are good for preserving strength (Delp, Statler, and Carroll 1995), but by nature do not allow for accurate characterization of the change in length induced. Instead, the surgeon is more often guided by feel and ascertains if the muscle is sufficiently taut in a given posture. This ideally would be made more precise by a force or stiffness measure. It may be possible to use intraoperative measures of shear wave speed as a proxy of tension in the operating room. Comparable work to address ligament tension via shear wave speed is ongoing and may ultimately enable intraoperative measures for balancing total knee replacements.

A final challenge is relating soft tissue treatment factors to outcomes. For this, there is tremendous need for reliable data that both characterize the treatment and provides objective measures for the outcome. More detailed surgical notes and intraoperative measures may enable better documentation of the treatments undertaken. Such data is particularly relevant for modelers who often require data as inputs to ensure their surgical simulations represent the procedures undertaken. In addition, objective outcome data is needed, particularly to ensure that outcome findings are transferrable across institutions. Currently, outcome data is largely based on the centers equipped with gait analysis laboratories to evaluate movement after treatment. While valuable, this approach leaves out the much smaller centers that are not equipped with the instrumentation needed to evaluate gait. The evolution of lower cost wearables and simpler video-based technologies for evaluating gait could enable many more centers to get objective outcomes, and thereby greatly extend the amount of data needed to relate treatment and outcomes. Such a large data approach is key to ultimately understanding the complex relationship between pathology, treatment, and gait that continues to challenge the many clinicians who are attempting to use gait disorders in individuals with CP.

The paradigm of evidence-based medicine is built upon the concept that clinical decision making based upon best evidence leads to the best outcomes. The best evidence is objective and quantitative; however, the existence of such evidence does not guarantee its utilization. The evidence-based medicine paradigm represents an effort to standardize care in clinical medicine, in which providers and patients are bound to a common knowledge base. Change in the direction of standardization of clinical practices is frequently incremental and proceeds through three stages. First, in the period of the proselytizers, the introduction of new technologies and techniques is enthusiastically embraced and promoted by a small number of visionaries, whose enthusiasm results in over-application of the new approaches and some number of poor outcomes, which offends the skeptical majority. Second, the period of the critical enthusiast, where clinical experience with the new paradigm leads to technological refinements and identification of appropriate indications. The final stage, the period of incorporation, occurs when familiarity and confidence with the new practices lead to acceptance and widespread utilization. Management of MTU dysfunction in children with CP is currently well into the period of the critical enthusiast. Improved understanding of pathoanatomy and pathophysiology of the MTU, modeling of soft tissue function (both physics and big data/machine learning-based), and commitment to objective, quantitative outcomes assessments in multiple domains should lead to the refinement of surgical indications and techniques. New techniques for teaching and learning, such as surgical simulation, patient-specific preoperative planning, and performing virtual surgery through digital twin technology should facilitate the knowledge translation that is necessary to proceed into the period of incorporation.

5-YEAR PRIORITIES

- **Fusing of models and data:** continue efforts to couple models, imaging, movement analysis, and outcomes to better understand the influence of myostatic contractures, spasticity, and selective motor control on mobility.
- **Assess dynamic muscle function:** leverage recent advances in shear wave tensiometry to directly evaluate dynamic muscle actions during gait analysis.
- **Enhance treatment precision:** evaluate use of imaging and intraoperative sensors to plan treatments and assess muscle tension during surgical procedures.
- **Objective documentation of treatments:** expand use of surgical notes, imaging, and objective measures to provide the data needed to evaluate models that can causally link treatment factors and outcomes.
- **Broader use of movement analysis:** evolution of low-cost wearables and simple video-based technologies should be leveraged to expand and extend the mobility data available to relate treatments with outcomes.

FUTURE NEEDS

- **Precision and consistency of interventions:** similar to the advancements in model-based preoperative planning for skeletal surgeries, there is a long-term need for technologies that can enable improved precision, efficiency in planning, and carrying out common, but currently non-standardized, soft tissue surgeries.
- **Knowledge translation:** new techniques for teaching and learning, such as surgical simulation, patient-specific preoperative planning, and performing virtual surgery through digital twin technology, are needed to facilitate the knowledge translation necessary to improve the acceptance and utilization of novel approaches to soft tissue treatments.
- **Scientific underpinnings:** improved understanding of pathoanatomy and pathophysiology of the MTU in CP and broad commitment to objective, quantitative outcome assessments are critical to long-term refinement of the approaches used for treating soft tissue impairments.

REFERENCES

Arnold AS, Liu MQ, Schwartz MH, Õunpuu S, Dias LS, Delp SL (2006) Do the hamstrings operate at increased muscle-tendon lengths and velocities after surgical lengthening? *Journal of Biomechanics* **39**: 1498–1506.

Arnold AS, Liu MQ, Schwartz MH, Õunpuu S, Delp SL (2006) The role of estimating muscle-tendon lengths and velocities of the hamstrings in the evaluation and treatment of crouch gait. *Gait and Posture* **23**: 273–281.

Athwal GS Ellis RE, Small CF, Pichora DR (2003) Computer-Assisted Distal Radius Osteotomy. *Journal of Hand Surgery* **28**: 951–958.

Barrett RS, Lichtwark GA (2010) Gross muscle morphology and structure in spastic cerebral palsy: a systematic review. *Developmental Medicine and Child Neurology* **52**: 794–804.

Bittmann MF, Lenhart RL, Schwartz MH, Novacheck TF, Hetzeld S, Thelenade DG (2018) How does patellar tendon advancement alter the knee extensor mechanism in children treated for crouch gait? *Gait Posture* **64**: 248–254.

Blum KP, Lamotte D'Incamps B, Zytnicki D, Ting LH (2017) Force encoding in muscle spindles during stretch of passive muscle. *PLoS Computational Biology* **13**: 1–24.

Brandon SCE, Thelen DG, Smith CR, Novacheck TF, Schwartz MH, Lenhart RL (2018) The coupled effects of crouch gait and patella alta on tibiofemoral and patellofemoral cartilage loading in children. *Gait Posture* **60**: 181–187.

Center for Disease Control and Prevention (2005) *Epidemiology and prevention of vaccine-preventable diseases*. Washington DC: Public Health Foundation.

Davids JR, Ounpuu S, DeLuca PA, Davis RB (2004) Optimization of walking ability of children with cerebral palsy. *Instructional course lectures* **53**: 511–522.

Davids JR, Oeffinger DJ, Bagley AM, Sison-Williamson M, Gorton G (2014) Relationship of strength, weight, age, and function in ambulatory children with cerebral palsy. *Journal of Pediatric Orthopaedics* **35**: 523–529.

Davids JR, Cung NQ, Sattler K, Boakes JL, Bagley AM (2019) Quantitative Assessment of Muscle Strength Following "slow" Surgical Lengthening of the Medial Hamstring Muscles in Children with Cerebral Palsy. *Journal of Pediatric Orthopaedics* **39**: e373–e379.

Davids JR, Rowan F, Davis RB (2007) Indications for orthoses to improve gait in children with cerebral palsy. *Journal of the American Academy of Orthopaedic Surgeons* **15**: 178–188.

Delp SL, Arnold AS, Speers RA, Moore CA (1996) Hamstrings and psoas lengths during normal and crouch gait: Implications for muscle-tendon surgery. *Journal of Orthopaedic Research* **14**: 144–151.

Delp SL, Anderson FC, Arnold AS et al. (2007) OpenSim: open-source software to create and analyze dynamic simulations of movement. *IEEE transactions on bio-medical engineering* **54**: 1940–1950.

Delp SL, Statler K, Carroll NC (1995) Preserving plantar flexion strength after surgical treatment for contracture of the triceps surae: A computer simulation study. *Journal of Orthopaedic Research* **13**: 96–104.

DeLuca PA, Ounpuu S, Davis RB, Walsh JH (1998) Effect of hamstring and Psoas lengthening on pelvic tilt in patients with spastic diplegic cerebral palsy. *Journal of Pediatric Orthopaedics* **18**: 712–718.

Dreher T, Buccoliero T, Wolf SI et al. (2012) Long-term results after gastrocnemius-soleus intramuscular aponeurotic recession as a part of multilevel surgery in spastic diplegic cerebral palsy. *Journal of Bone and Joint Surgery - Series A* **94**: 627–637.

Erdemir A, McLean S, Herzog W, van den Bogert AJ (2007) Model-based estimation of muscle forces exerted during movements. *Clinical Biomechanics* **22**: 131–154.

Falisse A, Bar-On L, Desloovere K, Jonkers I, De Groote F (2018) A spasticity model based on feedback from muscle force explains muscle activity during passive stretches and gait in children with cerebral palsy. *PLoS ONE* **13**: 1–20.

Firth GB, Passmore E, Sangeux M et al. (2013) Multilevel surgery for equinus gait in children with spastic diplegic cerebral palsy medium-term follow-up with gait analysis. *Journal of Bone and Joint Surgery - Series A* **95**: 931–938.

Graham HK, Rosenbaum P, Paneth N et al. (2016) Cerebral palsy. *Nature Reviews Disease Primers* **2**: 15082.

De Groote F, Blum KP, Horslen BC, Ting LH (2018) Interaction between muscle tone, short-range stiffness and increased sensory feedback gains explains key kinematic features of the pendulum test in spastic cerebral palsy: A simulation study. *PLoS ONE* **13**: 1–21.

Hicks JL, Uchida TK, Seth A, Rajagopal A, Delp SL (2015) Is my model good enough? Best practices for verification and validation of musculoskeletal models and simulations of human movement. *Journal of Biomechanical Engineering* **137**: 020905.

Jaspers RT, Brunner R, Riede UN, Huijing PA (2005) Healing of the aponeurosis during recovery from aponeurotomy: Morphological and histological adaptation and related changes in mechanical properties. *Journal of Orthopaedic Research* **23**: 266–273.

Keuler EM, Loegering IF, Martin JA, Roth JD, Thelen DG (2019) Shear Wave Predictions of Achilles Tendon Loading during Human Walking. *Scientific Reports* **9**: 1–9.

Lenhart RL, Brandon SC, Smith CR, Novacheck TF, Schwartz MH, Thelen DG (2017) Influence of patellar position on the knee extensor mechanism in normal and crouched walking. *Journal of Biomechanics* **51**: 1–7.

Martin JA, Brandon SCE, Keuler EM et al. (2018) Gauging force by tapping tendons. *Nature Communications* **9**: 1–9.

Mockford M, Caulton JM (2008) Systematic review of progressive strength training in children and adolescents with cerebral palsy who are ambulatory. *Pediatric Physical Therapy* **20**: 318–333.

Narayanan UG (2012) Management of children with ambulatory cerebral palsy: An evidence-based review. *Journal of Pediatric Orthopaedics* **32**: 172–181.

Novacheck TF, Gage JR (2007) Orthopedic management of spasticity in cerebral palsy. *Child's nervous system: ChNS: official journal of the International Society for Pediatric Neurosurgery* **23**: 1015–1031.

Oshinsky D (2006) *Polio: An American story.* New York: Oxford University Press.

Oskoui M, Coutinho F, Dykeman J, Jetté N, Pringsheim T (2013) An update on the prevalence of cerebral palsy: A systematic review and meta-analysis. *Developmental Medicine and Child Neurology* **55**: 509–519.

Pitto L, Kainz H, Falisse A et al. (2019) SimCP: A Simulation Platform to Predict Gait Performance Following Orthopedic Intervention in Children With Cerebral Palsy. *Frontiers in Neurorobotics* **13**: 54.

Rang M, Silver R, de la Garza J (1977) Cerebral palsy. In: Lovell WW, Winter RB, editors. *Pediatric Orthopaedics.* Philadelphia: JB Lippincott.

Robertson DGE, Caldwell GE, Hamill J, Kamen G, Whittlesey S (2013) *Research methods in biomechanics.* Champaign, IL: Human Kinetics.

Rose SA, DeLuca PA, Davis RB 3rd, Ounpuu S, Gage JR (1993) Kinematic and Kinetic Evaluation of the Ankle After Lengthening of the Gastrocnemius Fascia in Children with Cerebral Palsy. *Journal of Pediatric Orthopaedics* **13**: 727–732.

Rosenbaum P, Paneth N, Leviton A et al. (2007) A report: The definition and classification of cerebral palsy April 2006. *Developmental Medicine and Child Neurology* **49**: 480.

Schwartz MH, Rozumalski A, Novacheck TF (2014) Femoral derotational osteotomy: Surgical indications and outcomes in children with cerebral palsy. *Gait and Posture* **39**: 778–783.

Schwartz MH, Rozumalski A, Steele KM (2016) Dynamic motor control is associated with treatment outcomes for children with cerebral palsy. *Developmental Medicine and Child Neurology* **58**: 1139–1145.

Seireg A, Arvikar RJ (1973) A mathematical model for evaluation of forces in lower extremeties of the musculo-skeletal system. *Journal of Biomechanics* **6**: 313–326.

Seireg A, Arvikar RJ (1975) The prediction of muscular load sharing and joint forces in the lower extremities during walking. *Journal of Biomechanics* **8**: 89–102.

Seniorou M, Thompson N, Harrington M, Theologis T (2007) Recovery of muscle strength following multi-level orthopaedic surgery in diplegic cerebral palsy. *Gait and Posture* **26**: 475–481.

Sharrard WJW, Bernstein S (1972) Equinus Deformity In Cerebral Palsy. *The Journal of Bone and Joint Surgery* **54**: 272–276.

Shortland AP, Fry NR, McNee AE and Gough M (2009) Muscle structure and function in cerebral palsy, In Gage JR, Schwartz MH, Koop SE, Novacheck TF, editors, *The Identification and treatment Gait Problems in Cerebral Palsy,* London: MacKeith Press, pp 130–135.

Stout JL, Gage JR, Schwartz MH, Novacheck TF. (2008) Distal Femoral Extension Osteotomy and Patellar Tendon Advancement to Treat Persistent Crouch Gait in Cerebral Palsy. *The Journal of Bone and Joint Surgery-American Volume* **90**: 2470–2484.

Thelen DG (2003) Adjustment of muscle mechanics model parameters to simulate dynamic contractions in older adults. *Journal of Biomechanical Engineering* **125**: 70–77.

Tinney A, Khot A, Eizenberg N, Wolfe R, Graham HK (2014) Gastrocsoleus recession techniques: An anatomical and biomechanical study in human cadavers. *Bone and Joint Journal* **96**: 778–782.

Vaughan C, Davis B, O'Connor J (1992) *Dynamics of human gait* Cape Town: Kiboho Publishers.

Wiley ME, Damiano DL (2008) Lower-Extremity strength profiles in spastic cerebral palsy. *Developmental Medicine & Child Neurolog* **40**: 100–107.

Afterword

Tom Novacheck and I have been involved in the identification and treatment of mobility impairments in children diagnosed with cerebral palsy (CP) for over half a century combined. We have seen many changes in treatment philosophy, the technology used to assess patients, and the ways in which we measure and judge outcomes. Recently, we noticed – as did many others in the field – that progress seemed to be plateauing. We have asked ourselves, 'Is this the ceiling? Is this the best we can do for our patients? Or, are we missing something?' This awareness and these questions motivated us to try and identify gaps in our current understanding of patients, treatments, outcomes, and our underlying clinical 'model' of CP.

We chose a small, intensive, and focused symposium as a mechanism for probing these issues. We tried to assemble a team that represented a cross-section of age and experience, background, expertise, and personality. Our discussions reflected this diversity. There were great debates, many areas of unanimity, arguments, 'aha' moments, and times of deep reflection, frustration, and enlightenment. All of us felt enriched by the process, and our hope was to channel the tremendous energy of the event into this book. In the end, we felt that there were several common themes, among them: patient goals need more attention, outcomes have stagnated, the details of the underlying neurological impairments are still a mystery, and strong evidence for what we do is desperately needed.

In what must be a record for such undertakings, authors completed their chapters less than 4 months after we left Banff! This is a credit to the attendees, and also a reflection of the strong sense of purpose that emerged during the meeting.

Our hope is not that this document should form some sort of definitive 'last word', but rather it serves as a starting point. Perhaps it will motivate specific research projects. Perhaps it will stimulate additional efforts aimed at identifying critical priorities. Perhaps it will be used to support grant applications or other fundraising efforts. Maybe you agree with what we wrote. Maybe you think we have missed something critical. Whatever your response, we hope it results in action, and that the combined effort results in benefits for our patients.

Michael H Schwartz, PhD
2020

Index

NOTE: Tables, boxes and figures are denoted by a lowercase italicised t, b or f, followed by their respective number (ie. 17txx.x)

Other titles from Mac Keith Press www.mackeith.co.uk

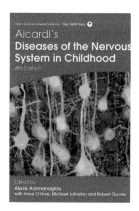

Aicardi's Diseases of the Nervous System in Childhood, 4th Edition

Alexis Arzimanoglou, Anne O'Hare, Michael V Johnston and Robert Ouvrier (Editors)

Clinics in Developmental Medicine
2018 ▪ 1524pp ▪ hardback ▪ 978-1-909962-80-4

This fourth edition retains the patient-focussed, clinical approach of its predecessors. The international team of editors and contributors has honoured the request of the late Jean Aicardi, that his book remain 'resolutely clinical', which distinguishes *Diseases of the Nervous System in Childhood* from other texts in the field. New edition completely updated and revised and now in full colour.

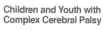

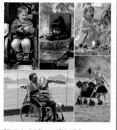

Children and Youth with Complex Cerebral Palsy: Care and Management

Laurie J. Glader and Richard D. Stevenson (Editors)

A Practical Guide from Mac Keith Press
2019 ▪ 404pp ▪ softback ▪ 978-1-909962-98-9

This is the first practical guide to explore management of the many medical comorbidities that children with complex CP face, including orthopaedics, mobility needs, cognition and sensory impairment, difficult behaviours, respiratory complications and nutrition, amongst others. Uniquely, contributors include children and parents, providing applied wisdom for family-centred care. Clinical Care Tools are provided to help guide clinicians and include a Medical Review Supplement, Equipment and Services Checklist and an ICF-Based Care: Goals and Management Form.

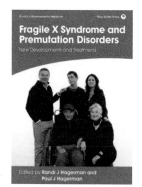

Fragile X Syndrome and Premutation Disorders: New Developments and Treatments

Randi J Hagerman and Paul J Hagerman (Editors)

Clinics in Developmental Medicine
2020 ▪ 176pp ▪ hardback ▪ 978-1-911612-37-7

Fragile X syndrome results from a gene mutation on the X-chromosome, which leads to various intellectual and developmental disabilities. *Fragile X Syndrome and Premutation Disorders* offers clinicians and families a multidisciplinary approach in order to provide the best possible care for patients with Fragile X. Unique features of the book include what to do when an infant or toddler is first diagnosed, the impact on the family and an international perspective on how different cultures perceive the syndrome.

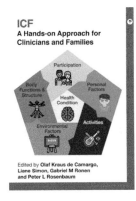

ICF: A Hands-on Approach for Clinicians and Families
Olaf Kraus de Camargo, Liane Simon, Gabriel M. Ronen and Peter L. Rosenbaum (Editors)

A Practical Guide from Mac Keith Press
2019 ▪ 192pp ▪ softback ▪ 978-1-911612-04-9

This accessible handbook introduces the World Health Organisation's International Classification of Functioning, Disability and Health (ICF) to professionals working with children with disabilities and their families. It contains an overview of the elements of the ICF but focusses on practical applications, including how the ICF framework can be used with children, families and carers to formulate health and management goals.

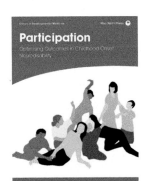

Participation: Optimising Outcomes in Childhood-Onset Neurodisability
Christine Imms and Dido Green (Editors)

Clinics in Developmental Medicine
2020 ▪ 288pp ▪ hardback ▪ 978-1-911612-17-9

This unique book focuses on enabling children and young people with neurodisability to participate in the varied life situations that form their personal, familial and cultural worlds. Chapters provide diverse examples of evidence-based practices and are enriched by scenarios and vignettes to engage and challenge the reader to consider how participation in meaningful activities might be optimised for individuals and their families. The book's practical examples aim to facilitate knowledge transfer, clinical application and service planning for the future.

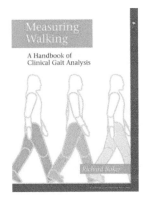

Measuring Walking: A Handbook of Clinical Gait Analysis
Richard Baker (Author)

A Practical Guide from Mac Keith Press
2013 ▪ 246pp ▪ softback ▪ 978-1-908316-66-0

This book is a practical guide to instrumented clinical gait analysis covering all aspects of routine service provision. It reinforces what is coming to be regarded as the conventional approach to clinical gait analysis. The book aims to describe the theoretical basis of gait analysis in conceptual terms. It then builds on this to give practical advice on how to perform the full spectrum of tasks that comprise contemporary clinical gait analysis.

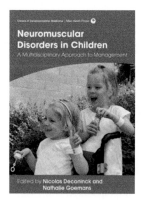

Neuromuscular Disorders in Children: A Multidisciplinary Approach to Management
Nicolas Deconinck and Nathalie Goemans (Editors)

Clinics in Developmental Medicine
2019 ▪ 468pp ▪ hardback ▪ 978-1-911612-09-4

Neuromuscular Disorders in Children: A Multidisciplinary Approach to Management critically reviews current evidence of management approaches in the field of neuromuscular disorders (NMDs) in children. Uniquely, the book focusses on assessment as the cornerstone of management and highlights the importance of a multidisciplinary approach.

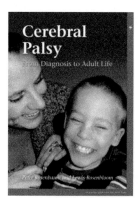

Cerebral Palsy: From Diagnosis to Adult Life
Peter L Rosenbaum and Lewis Rosenbloom (Editors)

A Practical Guide from Mac Keith Press
2012 ▪ 224pp ▪ softback ▪ 978-1-908316-50-9

This book has been designed to provide readers with an understanding of cerebral palsy as a developmental as well as a neurological condition. It details the nature of cerebral palsy, its causes and its clinical manifestations. Using clear, accessible language (supported by an extensive glossary) the authors have blended current science with metaphor to explain the biomedical underpinnings of cerebral palsy.

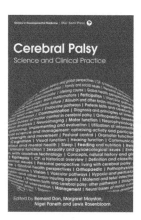

Cerebral Palsy: Science and Clinical Practice
Bernard Dan, Margaret Mayston, Nigel Paneth and Lewis Rosenbloom (Editors)

Clinics in Developmental Medicine
2015 ▪ 648pp ▪ hardback ▪ 978-1-909962-38-5

This landmark title considers all aspects of cerebral palsy from the causes to clinical problems and their implications for individuals. An international team of experts present a wide range of person-centred assessment approaches, including clinical evaluation, measurement scales, neuroimaging and gait analysis. The perspective of the book spans the lifelong course of cerebral palsy, taking into account worldwide differences in socio-economic and cultural factors. Full integrated colour, with extensive cross-referencing make this a highly attractive and useful reference.

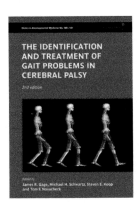

Nutrition and Neurodisability
Peter B. Sullivan, Guro L. Andersen and Morag J. Andrew (Editors)

A Practical Guide from Mac Keith Press
2020 ▪ 208pp ▪ softback ▪ 978-1-911612-26-1

Feeding difficulties are common in children with neurodisability and disorders of the central nervous system can affect the movements required for safe and efficient eating and drinking. This practical guide provides strategies for managing the range of nutritional problems faced by children with neurodevelopmental disability. The easily accessible information on aetiology, assessment and management is informed by a succinct review of current evidence and guidelines to inform best practice.

Identification and Treatment of Gait Problems in Cerebral Palsy, 2nd Edition
James R. Gage, Michael H Schwartz, Steven E Koop and Tom F Novacheck (Editors)

Clinics in Developmental Medicine
2009 ▪ 660pp ▪ hardback ▪ 978-1-898683-65-0

The only book to deal specifically with the treatment of gait problems in cerebral palsy, this comprehensive, multi-disciplinary volume is invaluable for all those working in the field of cerebral palsy and gait. The first part is designed to help the reader evaluate and understand a child with cerebral palsy. The second is a comprehensive overview of management. It emphasizes the most fundamental concept of treatment: manage the child's neurologic dysfunction first and then address the skeletal and muscular consequences of that dysfunction.

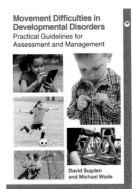

Movement Difficulties in Developmental Disorders
David Sugden and Michael Wade (Authors)

A Practical Guide from Mac Keith Press
2019 ▪ 240pp ▪ softback ▪ 978-1-909962-95-8

This book presents the latest evidence-based approaches to assessing and managing movement disorders in children. Uniquely, children with developmental coordination disorder (DCD) and children with movement difficulties as a co-occurring secondary characteristic of another development disorder, including ADHD, ASD, and Dyslexia, are discussed. It will prove a valuable guide for anybody working with children with movement difficulties, including clinicians, teachers and parents.